P9-CMX-482

PHYSICAL EXAMINATION

& Health Assessment

PHYSICAL EXAMINATION & Health Assessment

Fifth Edition

Carolyn Jarvis, PhD, APN, CNP
Adjunct Associate Professor of Nursing
School of Nursing
Illinois Wesleyan University
and
Family Nurse Practitioner
Chestnut Health Systems
Bloomington, Illinois

Original Illustrations by Pat Thomas, CMI, FAMI
Oak Park, Illinois

Assessment Photographs by Kevin Strandberg
Professor of Art
Illinois Wesleyan University
Bloomington, Illinois

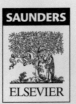

SAUNDERS

ELSEVIER

SAUNDERS
ELSEVIER

11830 Westline Industrial Drive
St. Louis, Missouri 63146

Pocket Companion for Physical Examination and Health Assessment

ISBN: 978-1-4160-3854-2

Copyright © 2008, 2004, 2000, 1996, 1993 by Saunders, and imprint of Elsevier Inc.

NOTICE

Pharmacology is an ever-changing field. Standard safety precautions must be followed, but as new research and clinical experience broaden our knowledge, changes in treatment and drug therapy may become necessary or appropriate. Readers are advised to check the most current product information provided by the manufacturer of each drug to be administered to verify the recommended dose, the method and duration of administration, and contraindications. It is the responsibility of the licensed prescriber, relying on experience and knowledge of the patient, to determine dosages and the best treatment for each individual patient. Neither the publisher nor the author assumes any liability for any injury and/or damage to persons or property arising from this publication.

Previous editions copyrighted 2004, 2000, 1996, 1993

Library of Congress Control Number: 2007936010

Executive Editor: Robin Carter
Developmental Editor: Deanna Davis
Publishing Services Manager: Jeff Patterson
Project Manager: Amy Rickles
Cover Designer: Paula Catalano
Text Designer: Paula Catalano

Working together to grow
libraries in developing countries

www.elsevier.com | www.bookaid.org | www.sabre.org

ELSEVIER   BOOK AID International   Sabre Foundation

Printed in Canada

Last digit is the print number: 9 8 7 6 5 4 3 2

About the Author

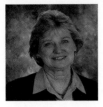

Carolyn Jarvis received her BSN cum laude from the University of Iowa, her MSN from Loyola University (Chicago), and her PhD from the University of Illinois in Chicago, with a research interest in the physiologic effect of alcohol on the cardiovascular system. She has taught physical assessment and critical care nursing at Rush University (Chicago), University of Missouri (Columbia), and University of Illinois (Urbana), and she has taught physical assessment, pharmacology, and pathophysiology at Illinois Wesleyan University (Bloomington).

Dr. Jarvis is a recipient of the University of Missouri's Superior Teaching Award and has taught physical assessment to thousands of baccalaureate students, graduate students, and nursing professionals, has held 150 continuing education seminars, and is the author of numerous articles and textbook contributions. Dr. Jarvis has maintained a clinical practice in advanced practice roles—first as a cardiovascular clinical specialist in various critical care settings and as a certified family nurse practitioner in primary care. She is currently an associate professor at Illinois Wesleyan University, a nurse practitioner at Chestnut Health Systems, Bloomington, Illinois, and is licensed as an advanced practice nurse in the state of Illinois.

Preface

The fifth edition of *Pocket Companion for Physical Examination and Health Assessment*, in full-color throughout, is designed for two groups—those who need a practical clinical reference and those acquiring beginning assessment skills.

First, the *Pocket Companion* is intended as an adjunct to Jarvis' *Physical Examination and Health Assessment*, 5th ed. The *Pocket Companion* is a memory prompt for those who have studied physical assessment and wish a reminder when in the clinic. The *Pocket Companion* has all the essentials: health history points, exam steps for each body system, normal versus abnormal findings, heart sounds, lung sounds, neurologic checks. *The Pocket Companion* is useful when you forget a step in the exam sequence, when you wish to be sure your assessment is complete, when you need to review the findings that are normal versus abnormal, or when you are faced with an unfamiliar technique or a new clinical area. Its portable size and binding make it perfect for a lab coat pocket or community health bag.

Second, the *Pocket Companion*, 5th ed. is an independent primer of basic assessment skills. It is well suited to programs offering a beginning assessment course covering well people of all ages. The *Pocket Companion* has the complete steps to perform a health history and physical examination on a well person. It includes pertinent developmental content for pediatric, pregnant, and aging adult patients. Although the description of each exam step is stated concisely, there is enough information given to study and learn exam techniques. However, since there is no room in the *Pocket Companion* for theories, principles, or detailed explanations, students using the *Pocket Companion* as a beginning text must have a thorough didactic presentation of assessment methods as well as tutored practice.

The *Pocket Companion*, 5th ed., is revised and updated to match the revision of the parent text, *Physical Examination and Health Assessment*, 5th ed., including new examination photos and new full color art.

For those times when readers need detailed coverage of a particular technique or finding, it is easily found through numerous cross-references to pages *in Physical Examination and Health Assessment*, 5th ed.

As you thumb through the *Pocket Companion,* note these features:

- Health history and exam steps are concise yet complete.
- Method of examination is clear, orderly, and easy to follow.
- Abnormal findings are described briefly in a column adjacent to the normal range of findings.
- Tables are presented at the end of chapters to fully illustrate important information.
- Selected Cross-Cultural Care information highlights this important aspect of a health assessment.
- Nursing diagnoses are provided fully for each region or system being assessed.
- Developmental content includes age-specific information for pediatric, pregnant, and aging adult groups.
- Summary checklists for each chapter form a cue card of exam steps to remember.

- Integration of the complete physical examination is presented in Chapter 20.
- Sample Recording in Chapter 20 illustrates the documentation of normal findings.

- Selected artwork from *Physical Examination and Health Assessment*, 5th ed., illustrates the pertinent anatomy.

CAROLYN JARVIS

Acknowledgments

My thanks extend to Robin Carter, Executive Editor, Nursing, for her strong support and thorough team leadership in this project. Thanks to Deanna Davis, Developmental Editor, for her skillful effort and determination in this project from start to finish. I am grateful to Amy Rickles, Project Manager, and to Jeff Patterson, Publishing Services Manager, for their attentive monitoring of all stages of the *Pocket Companion*. Finally, thanks to Caitlin Zindars for helping to proofread at all stages.

CAROLYN JARVIS

Contents

Chapter One

The Interview and the Health History

The health history is important in beginning to identify the person's health strengths and problems and as a bridge to the next step in data collection, the physical examination.

The health history collects **subjective data,** what the person says about himself or herself. This is the first and the best chance a person has to tell you what *he* or *she* perceives his or her health state to be.

EXTERNAL FACTORS

Ensure Privacy. Aim for geographic privacy—a private room. If geographic privacy is not available, the "psychological privacy" afforded by curtained partitions may suffice as long as the person feels sure no one can overhear the conversation or interrupt.

Refuse Interruptions. You need this time to concentrate and to establish rapport.

Physical Environment

- Set the room temperature at a comfortable level.
- Provide sufficient lighting.
- Reduce noise.
- Remove distracting objects.
- Maintain the distance between you and the patient at 4 to 5 feet (twice an arm's length).
- Arrange equal-status seating. Both of you should be comfortably seated at eye level. Avoid sitting behind a desk or bedside table placed so that it looks like a barrier.
- Avoid standing.

There are three phases to each interview: an introduction, a working phase, and a termination (or closing).

INTRODUCING THE INTERVIEW

Address the patient using his or her surname. Introduce yourself and state your role in the agency (if you are a student, say so). If you are gathering a complete history, give the reason for this interview.

THE WORKING PHASE

The working phase is the data-gathering phase. It involves your questions to the patient and your responses to what the patient has said. There are two types of questions: open-ended and closed (or direct). Each type has a different place and function in the interview.

Open-Ended Questions

An open-ended question asks for narrative information. It states the topic to be discussed, but only in general terms. Use it to begin the interview, to introduce a new section of questions, and whenever the person introduces a new topic. Examples are "Tell me why you have come here today" and "What brings you to the hospital?"

Closed or Direct Questions

Closed or direct questions ask for specific information. They elicit a one- or two-word answer, a "yes" or "no," or a forced choice. Use direct questions after the person's narrative to fill in any details he or she may have omitted. Also use direct questions when you need many specific facts, such as when asking about past health problems or during the review of systems.

Responses

As the person talks, your role is to encourage free expression but not let him or her wander. The following responses help you gather data without cutting the person off.

Facilitation. Your facilitative response encourages the patient to say more, to continue with the story, e.g., "mm-hmm," "go on," "continue," "uh-huh," or simply nodding.

Silence. Your silence communicates that the patient has time to think, to organize what he or she wishes to say without interruption from you. Silence also gives you a chance to observe the person unobtrusively and to note nonverbal cues.

Reflection. A reflective response echoes the patient's own words. Reflection involves repeating part of what the person has just said. It focuses further attention on a specific phrase and helps the person continue in his or her own way.

Empathy. An empathic response recognizes a feeling and puts it into words. It names the feeling and allows its expression. When you use an empathic response, the patient feels accepted and can deal with the feeling openly. Empathic responses include saying, "This must be very hard for you" and just placing your hand on the person's arm.

Clarification. Use the clarification response when the patient's word choice is ambiguous or confusing, e.g., "Tell me what you mean by 'tired blood.'"

Confrontation. In this case, you have observed a certain action, feeling, or statement, and you now focus the person's attention on it. This can focus on a discrepancy: "You say it doesn't hurt, but when I touch you here, you grimace." It can also focus on the patient's affect: "You look sad" or "You sound angry."

Interpretation. An interpretive response is based not on direct observation (as is confrontation) but on your inference or conclusion. Interpretation links events, makes associations, or implies cause: "It seems that every time you feel the stomach pain, you have had some kind of stress in your life."

Explanation. With these statements, you share factual and objective information. This may be for orientation to the agency setting: "Your dinner comes at 5:30 PM"; or it may be to explain cause: "The reason you cannot eat or drink before your blood test is that the food will change the test results."

Summary. This is a final review of what you understand the patient has said. It condenses the facts and presents a survey of how you perceive the patient's health problem or need.

CLOSING THE INTERVIEW

The meeting should end gracefully. To ease into the closing, ask the patient, "Is there anything else you would like to mention?" Give the person a final opportunity for self-expression. Then give a summary or recapitulation of what you have learned during the interview. This is a final statement of what you and the patient agree his or her health state to be.

TEN TRAPS OF INTERVIEWING

Nonproductive, defeating verbal messages are messages that restrict the patient's response. They are obstacles to obtaining complete data and to establishing rapport.

1. Providing False Reassurance. Such statements as, "Now don't worry,

I'm sure you will be all right" are courage builders that relieve *your* anxiety and give you a false sense of having provided comfort. For the patient, however, these statements close off communication. They trivialize anxiety and effectively deny further discussion.

2. Giving Unwanted Advice. A person describes a problem to you, ending with, "What would you do?" If you answer, "If I were you, I'd . . . ," you have shifted the accountability for decision-making from the patient to you. The person has not worked out his or her own solution and has learned nothing about himself or herself.

3. Using Authority. "Your doctor/nurse knows best" is a response that promotes dependency and inferiority.

4. Using Avoidance Language. People use euphemisms, such as "passed on," to avoid reality or to hide their feelings.

5. Engaging in Distancing. Distancing is the use of impersonal speech to put space between a threat and oneself, e.g., "There is a lump in *the* left breast."

6. Using Professional Jargon. Use of jargon sounds exclusionary and paternalistic. You need to adjust your vocabulary to the patient but should avoid sounding condescending.

7. Using Leading or Biased Questions. Asking such questions as, "You don't smoke, do you?" implies that one answer is "better" than another.

8. Talking Too Much. Some examiners associate helpfulness with how much they talk. They think they have met the patient's needs. Just the opposite is true.

9. Interrupting. Often, when you think you know what the person will say, you interrupt and cut him or her off.

10. Using "Why" Questions. The adult's use of "why" questions usually implies blame and condemnation, and puts the patient on the defensive.

Nonverbal Skills

Nonverbal messages that are productive and enhancing to the relationship are those that show attentiveness and unconditional acceptance. Defeating and nonproductive nonverbal behaviors are those of inattentiveness, authority, and superiority (Table 1–1).

TABLE 1–1	Nonverbal Behaviors of the Interviewer	
Positive	**Negative**
Appropriate professional appearance	Appearance objectionable to patient
Equal-status seating	Standing
Close placement to patient	Sitting behind desk, far away, turned away
Relaxed open posture	Tense posture
Leaning slightly toward person	Slouched back
Occasional facilitation gestures	Critical or distracting gestures: pointing finger, clenched fist, finger-tapping, foot-swinging, looking at watch
Facial animation, interest	Bland expression, yawning, tight mouth
Appropriate smiling	Frowning, lip biting
Appropriate eye contact	Shifting eyes, avoiding eye contact, focusing on notes
Moderate tone of voice	Strident, high-pitched tone
Moderate rate of speech	Rate too slow or too fast
Appropriate touch	Too frequent or inappropriate touch

THE HEALTH HISTORY: THE ADULT

Biographical Data

This information includes name, address, telephone number, age, birth date, birthplace, sex, marital status, race, ethnic origin, and occupation, usual and present.

Source of History

The history may be provided by the patient himself or herself or by a substitute.

Reason for Seeking Care

This is a brief spontaneous statement in the patient's own words that describes the reason for the visit.

Present Health or History of Present Illness

This is a chronologic record of the reason for seeking care, from the time of the onset of the symptoms until now. Start when the person first noticed the symptoms and work forward to the present. Your final summary of any symptom the patient has should include these *critical characteristics,* organized into the mnemonic PQRSTU to help remember all the points.

P. **Provocative or palliative.** What brings it on? What were you doing when you first noticed it? What makes it better? Worse?
Q. **Quality or quantity.** How does it look, feel, sound? How intense/severe is it?
R. **Region or radiation.** Where is it? Does it spread anywhere?
S. **Severity scale.** How bad is it (on a scale ranging from 1 to 10)? Is it getting better, worse, staying the same?
T. **Timing.** Onset—Exactly when did it first occur? Duration—How long did it last? Frequency—How often does it occur?
U. **Understand** *patient's perception* of the problem. What do you think it means?

Past Health

Childhood Illnesses. Measles, mumps, rubella, chickenpox, pertussis, strep throat, rheumatic fever, scarlet fever, and poliomyelitis.

Accidents or Injuries

Serious or Chronic Illnesses. Diabetes, hypertension, heart disease, sickle-cell anemia, cancer, and seizure disorder.

Hospitalizations and Operations

Obstetric History. The number of pregnancies (gravidity), number of deliveries in which the fetus reached viability (parity), and number of incomplete pregnancies or abortions. This is recorded as G_P_Ab_ (e.g., G3 P2 Ab1).

Immunizations. All childhood immunizations (measles/mumps/rubella, poliomyelitis, diphtheria/pertussis/tetanus, hepatitis B, hepatitis A in selected areas, *Haemophilus influenzae* type b, and pneumococcal vaccine). Also note the last tetanus immunization, last tuberculosis skin test, and last flu shot.

Last Examination Date. The most recent physical, dental, vision, hearing, electrocardiogram, and chest x-ray examinations.

Allergies. Medication, food, environmental agent. Note reaction.

Current Medications. All prescription and over-the-counter medications, including laxatives, vitamins, birth control pills, aspirin, and antacids.

Family History

The age and health or the age and cause of death of blood relatives, such as parents, grandparents, and siblings. The age and health of spouse and children. Specifically, any family history of heart disease, high blood pressure, stroke, diabetes, blood disorders, cancer, sickle-cell anemia, arthritis, allergies, obesity, alcoholism, mental illness, seizure disorder, kidney disease, or tuberculosis. Construct a family tree, or genogram, to show this information clearly and concisely (Fig. 1–1, p. 6).

Review of Systems

General Overall Health State. Present weight (gain or loss, period of time, by diet or other factors), fatigue, weakness or malaise, fever, chills, and sweats or night sweats.

Skin. History of skin disease (eczema, psoriasis, hives), pigment or color change, change in mole, excessive dryness or moisture, pruritus, excessive bruising, and rash or lesion.

Health Promotion. Amount of sun exposure.

Hair. Recent loss, change in texture.

Nails. Change in shape, color, or brittleness.

Head. Unusually frequent or severe headache, any head injury, dizziness (syncope), or vertigo.

Eyes. Difficulty with vision (decreased acuity, blurring, blind spots); eye pain; diplopia (double vision); redness or swelling; watering or discharge; and glaucoma or cataracts.

Health Promotion. Glasses or contact lens use, last vision check or glaucoma test, and ways of coping with vision loss.

Ears. Earaches, infections, discharge and its characteristics, tinnitus, or vertigo.

Health Promotion. Hearing loss, hearing aid use, effect of hearing loss on daily life, exposure to environ-

mental noise, and method of cleaning ears.

Nose and Sinuses. Discharge and its characteristics, unusually frequent or severe colds, any sinus pain, nasal obstruction, nosebleeds, allergies or hay fever, or change in sense of smell.

Mouth and Throat. Mouth pain, frequent sore throat, bleeding gums, toothache, lesion in mouth or tongue, dysphagia, hoarseness or voice change, or altered taste. History of tonsillectomy.

Health Promotion. Pattern of daily dental care, use of prosthesis (dentures, bridge), and last dental checkup.

Neck. Pain, limitation of motion, lumps or swelling, enlarged or tender nodes, or goiter.

Breast. Pain, lump, nipple discharge, rash, or breast disease.

Health Promotion. Breast self-examination method and frequency, last mammogram.

Axilla. Tenderness, lump or swelling, or rash.

Respiratory System. History of lung diseases (asthma, emphysema, bronchitis, pneumonia, tuberculosis); chest pain with breathing; wheezing or noisy breathing; shortness of breath; how much activity produces shortness of breath; cough; sputum (color, amount); hemoptysis; and toxin or pollution exposure.

Cardiovascular System. Precordial or retrosternal pain, palpitation, cyanosis, dyspnea on exertion (specify amount of exertion), orthopnea, paroxysmal nocturnal dyspnea, nocturia, edema, and history of heart murmur, hypertension, coronary artery disease, or anemia.

Peripheral Vascular System. Coldness, numbness and tingling, swelling of legs (time of day and activity), discoloration in hands or feet, varicose veins or complications, intermittent claudication, thrombophlebitis, or ulcers.

Drawing Your Family Tree
- Make a list of all of your family members.
- Use this sample family tree as a guide to draw your own family tree.
- Write your name at the top of your paper and date you drew your family tree.
- In place of the words father, mother etc., write the names of your family members.
- When possible, draw your brothers and sister and your parents' brothers and sisters starting from oldest to youngest, going from left to right across the paper.
- If dates of birth or ages are not known, then estimate or guess ("50s," "late 60s")

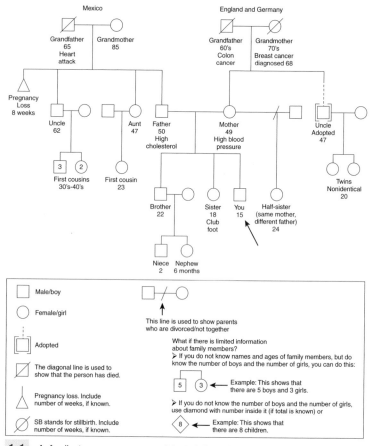

1–1   A family tree, or genogram. Adapted from the American Society of Human Genetics, www.ashg.org, 2004.

Health Promotion. Amount of long-term sitting or standing, habit of crossing legs at the knees, use of support hose.

Gastrointestinal System. Appetite; food intolerance; dysphagia; heartburn; indigestion; pain (associated with eating); other abdominal pain; pyrosis (esophageal and stomach burning sensation with sour eructation); nausea and vomiting (character); vomiting blood; history of abdominal disease (ulcer, liver or gallbladder, jaundice, appendicitis, colitis); flatulence; frequency of bowel movements (any recent change); stool characteristics; constipation or diarrhea; black stools; rectal bleeding; or rectal conditions (hemorrhoids, fistula).

Urinary System. Frequency or urgency; nocturia (recent change), dysuria, polyuria, or oliguria; hesitancy or straining; narrowed stream; urine color (cloudy or presence of blood), incontinence; history of urinary disease (kidney disease, kidney stones, urinary tract infections, prostate disease); or pain in flank, groin, suprapubic region, or low back.

Health Promotion. Use of Kegel exercises after childbirth, measures to avoid or treat urinary tract infections.

Male Genital System. Penile or testicular pain, sores or lesions, penile discharge, lumps, or hernia.

Health Promotion. Testicular self-examination method and frequency.

Female Genital System. Menstrual history (age at menarche, last menstrual period, cycle and duration, amenorrhea or menorrhagia, premenstrual pain or dysmenorrhea, intermenstrual spotting); vaginal itching; discharge and its characteristics; age at menopause; menopausal signs or symptoms; or postmenopausal bleeding.

Health Promotion. Last gynecologic checkup and last Papanicolaou smear.

Sexual Health. Current sexual activity, level of sexual satisfaction of patient and partner, dyspareunia (for female), changes in erection or ejaculation (for male), use of contraceptive and satisfaction with it, any known or suspected contact with a partner who has a sexually transmitted disease (gonorrhea, herpes, chlamydia, venereal warts, HIV/AIDS, or syphilis).

Musculoskeletal System. History of arthritis or gout. Joint pain, stiffness, swelling (location, migratory nature), deformity, limitation of motion, or noise with joint motion. Muscle pain, cramps, weakness, gait problems, or problems with coordinated activities. Other pain (location and radiation to extremities), stiffness, limitation of motion, or history of back pain or disc disease.

Health Promotion. Distance walked per day; effect of limited range of motion on daily activities, such as grooming, feeding, toileting, or dressing; and use of mobility aids.

Neurologic System. History of seizure disorder, stroke, fainting, or blackouts. Motor function: any weakness, tic or tremor, paralysis or coordination problems. Sensory function: any numbness and tingling (paresthesia). Cognitive function: any memory disorder (recent or distant, disorientation). Mental status: nervousness, mood change, depression, or history of mental health dysfunction or hallucinations.

Hematologic System. Bleeding of skin or mucous membranes, excessive bruising, lymph node swelling, exposure to toxic agents or radiation, or blood transfusion and reactions.

Endocrine System. History of diabetes or diabetic symptoms (polyuria, polydipsia, polyphagia); history of thyroid disease; intolerance to heat and cold; change in skin pigmentation or texture; excessive sweating; relationship between appetite and weight; abnormal hair distribution; nervousness; tremors; or need for hormone therapy.

Functional Assessment (Activities of Daily Living)

Functional assessment measures a person's self-care ability in the areas of physical health; activities of daily living (ADLs), such as bathing, dressing, toileting, and eating; instrumental activities of daily living (IADLs), which are those needed for independent living, such as housekeeping, shopping, and cooking; nutritional status; social relationships and resources; self-concept and coping; and home environment. These questions provide data on the lifestyle and type of living environment to which the person is accustomed.

Self-Esteem/Self-Concept. Education (last grade completed, other significant training); financial status (income adequate for lifestyle and/or health concerns); and values and belief system (religious practices and perception of personal strengths).

Activity/Exercise. A daily profile reflecting usual daily activities. Ability to perform ADLs—independent or needs assistance. Ability to tolerate activity or to use prostheses or mobility aids. Leisure activities enjoyed and exercise pattern (type, amount per day or week, warm-up session, body's response to exercise).

Sleep/Rest. Sleep patterns, any sleep aids, or daytime naps.

Nutrition/Elimination. All food and beverages taken over the last 24 hours: "Is that menu typical?" Eating habits and current appetite. "Who buys food and prepares food? Are finances adequate for food? Who is present at mealtimes?" Any food allergy or intolerance. Daily intake of caffeine (coffee, tea, cola drinks).

Interpersonal Relationships/ Resources. Social roles: "What's your role in your family? How would you say you get along with family, friends, and co-workers?" Support systems composed of family and significant others: "To whom could you go for support with a problem at work, with your health, or a personal problem?" Amount of time spent alone: "Is this pleasurable or isolating?"

Coping and Stress Management. Stresses in life now and in the past year, any change in lifestyle or any current stress, and any steps taken to relieve stress.

Personal Habits. Alcohol: "When was your last drink of alcohol? How much did you drink that time? Have you ever had a drinking problem?" Smoking: "Do you smoke? At what age did you start? How many packs do you smoke per day? How many years have you smoked?" Street drugs: "Have you ever tried any drugs such as marijuana, cocaine, amphetamines, or bar-

biturates? How often do you use these drugs? How has usage affected your work or social relationships?"

Environment/Hazards. Housing and neighborhood (live alone, know neighbors, safety of area, adequate heat and utilities, access to transportation, involved in community services); and environmental health (hazards in workplace, hazards at home, use of seatbelts, geographic or occupational exposures, travel or residence in other countries).

Intimate Partner Violence. "How are things at home? Do you feel safe?" If the person responds to feeling unsafe, follow up with, "Have you ever been emotionally or physically abused by your partner or someone important to you? Within the last year, have you been hit, slapped, kicked, pushed or shoved, or otherwise physically hurt by your partner or ex-partner? If yes, by whom? Number of times? Does your partner ever force you into having sex? Are you afraid of your partner or ex-partner?"

Occupational Health. "Please describe your job. Ever worked with any health hazard, asbestos, inhalants, chemicals, repetitive motion? Wear or use any protective equipment? Any work programs to monitor your exposure? Any health problems now you think are related to work? What do you like or dislike about your work?"

Perception of Health

"How do you define health? How do you view your situation now? What are your concerns? What do you think will happen in the future? What are your health goals? What do you expect from us as nurses, physicians, other health care providers?"

For more information on the health history of infants and children, older adults, and cultural assessment, see Jarvis: *Physical Examination and Health Assessment,* 5th ed., pp. 78–96.

Chapter Two

Mental Status

Mental status is a person's emotional and cognitive functioning. Optimal functioning aims toward simultaneous life satisfaction in work, in caring relationships, and within the self.

Mental status cannot be scrutinized directly like the characteristics of skin or heart sounds. Its functioning is *inferred* through assessment of an individual's behaviors:

Consciousness: awareness of one's own existence, feelings, and thoughts and awareness of the environment

Language: using the voice to communicate one's thoughts and feelings

Mood and affect: both of these elements deal with prevailing feelings; mood is a prolonged display of feelings that colors the whole emotional life, while affect is a temporary expression of feelings

Orientation: awareness of the objective world in relation to the self

Attention: the power of concentration, the ability to focus on one specific thing without being distracted

Memory: the ability to note and store experiences and perceptions for later recall; *recent* memory evokes day-to-day events, and *remote* memory brings up many years' worth of experiences

Abstract reasoning: pondering of a deeper meaning beyond the concrete and literal

Thought process: the *way* a person thinks, the logical train of thought

Thought content: *what* a person thinks; specific ideas, beliefs, and use of words

Perceptions: awareness of objects through any of the five senses

THE MENTAL STATUS EXAMINATION

The full mental status examination is a systematic check of emotional and cognitive functioning. The steps described here, though, rarely need to be taken in their entirety. Usually, you can assess mental status through the context of the health history interview. During that time, keep in mind the four main headings of mental status assessment:

Appearance
Behavior
Cognition
Thought processes

or A, B, C, T.

In every mental status examination, note these factors from the health history that could affect your interpretation of findings:

- Any known illnesses or health problems, such as alcoholism or chronic renal disease
- Current medications whose side effects can cause confusion or depression
- The usual educational and behavioral level; note that factor as the normal baseline, and do not expect performance on the mental status examination to exceed it
- Responses to personal history questions, indicating current stress, social interaction patterns, sleep habits, drug and alcohol use

Appearance

Posture and Position. Posture is erect, and position is relaxed.

Body Movements. Voluntary, deliberate, coordinated, and smooth and even.

Dress. Appropriate for setting, season, age, gender, and social group. Clothing fits and is put on appropriately.

Grooming and Hygiene. The person is clean and well groomed; hair is neat and clean; women have moderate or no make-up; men are clean shaven or the beard or mustache is well groomed. Nails are clean (though some jobs leave nails chronically dirty). Note that a disheveled appearance in a previously well-groomed person is significant. Use care in interpreting clothing that is disheveled, bizarre, or in poor repair because this sometimes may reflect the person's economic status or a deliberate fashion trend.

Behavior

Level of Consciousness. The person is alert, aware of stimuli from the environment and within the self, and responds appropriately (Table 2–1 on pp. 12-13).

Facial Expression. The look is appropriate to the situation and changes appropriately with the topic. There is comfortable eye contact unless precluded by cultural norm (e.g., Native American).

Speech. *Quality:* The person makes laryngeal sounds effortlessly and shares conversation appropriately.

The *pace* of the conversation is moderate, and stream of talking is fluent.

Articulation (ability to form words) is clear and understandable.

Word choice is effortless and appropriate to educational level. The person completes sentences, occasionally pausing to think.

Mood/Affect. Determine this by body language and facial expression and by asking, "How do you feel today" or "How do you usually feel?" The mood should be appropriate to the person's place and condition and should change appropriately with topics. The person is willing to cooperate with you.

Cognitive Functions

Orientation. You can discern orientation through the course of the interview. Assess:

Time: day of week, date, year, season
Place: where person lives, present location, type of building, name of city and state
Person: own name, age, who examiner is, type of worker

Many hospitalized people normally have trouble with the exact date but are fully oriented to other items.

Attention Span. Check the person's ability to concentrate by noting whether he or she completes a thought without wandering. Note any distractibility or difficulty attending to you, or give a series of directions to follow and note the correct sequence of behaviors. Be aware that attention span commonly is impaired in people who are anxious, fatigued, or drug intoxicated.

Recent Memory. Assess recent memory in the context of the interview by the 24-hour diet recall.

Remote Memory. In the context of the interview, ask the person verifiable past events, e.g., past health, first job, birthday and anniversary dates, and historic events.

Judgment. To assess judgment in the context of the interview, note what the person says about job plans, social or family obligations, and plans for the future. Also ask the person to describe the rationale for personal health care and how he or she decided about complying with prescribed health regimens. The person's actions and decisions should be realistic.

Thought Processes and Perceptions

Thought Processes. Ask yourself whether the patient makes sense and whether you can follow what he or she is saying. The way a person thinks should be logical, goal directed, coherent, and relevant. The person should complete a thought.

Thought Content. *What* the person says should be consistent and logical.

Perceptions. The person should be consistently aware of reality. His or her perceptions should be congruent with yours. Ask the following questions:

- "How do people treat you?"
- "Do other people talk about you?"
- "Do you feel as if you are being watched, followed, or controlled?"
- "Is your imagination very active?"
- "Have you heard your name when alone?"

Screen for Suicidal Thoughts. When the person expresses feelings of sadness, hopelessness, or despair or grief, it is important to assess any possible risk of physical self-harm. Begin with more general questions. If you hear affirmative answers, continue with more specific questions:

- "Have you ever felt so blue you thought of hurting yourself?"
- "Do you feel like hurting yourself now?"
- "Do you have a plan to hurt yourself?"
- "What would happen if you were dead?"
- "How would other people react if you were dead?"

Do not skip these questions if you have the slightest hint that they are appropriate. You may be the only health professional to pick up clues to suicide risk. You are responsible for encouraging the person to talk about suicidal thoughts. Sometimes you cannot prevent a suicide when someone really wishes to kill himself or herself. Most people are ambivalent, however, and you can buy time, so that the person can be helped to find an alternate solution to the situation.

Supplemental Mental Status Examination

The MiniMental State Examination (MMSE) is a simplified scored form of the cognitive functions of the mental status examination (Folstein, et al., 1975). It is quick and easy, includes a standard set of only 11 questions, and requires only 5 to 10 minutes to administer. It is useful for both initial and serial measurement, so you can demonstrate worsening or improvement of cognition over time and with treatment. The MMSE concentrates only on cognitive functioning, not on mood or thought processes. It is a valid detector of organic disease and thus is a good screening tool for detecting dementia and delirium (Fig. 2–1). For a full copy of the MMSE, see Jarvis: *Physical Examination and Health Assessment,* 5th ed., p. 104.

The maximum score on the test is 30; people with normal mental status average 27. Scores that occur with dementia and delirium are 18–23, mild cognitive impairment; 0–17, severe cognitive impairment.

For more information on abnormalities of mood and affect, delirium and dementia, substance use disorders, schizophrenia, mood disorders, and anxiety disorders, see Jarvis: *Physical Examination and Health Assessment,* 5th ed., pp. 108–118.

REGIONAL WRITE-UP—MENTAL STATUS EXAMINATION

Patient _____ Age _____ Sex _____ Occupation _____

Date _____

Examiner _____

Mental Status

(Before testing, tell the person the four words you want him or her to remember and to recall in a few minutes, for the Four Unrelated Words Test.)

1. Appearance

Posture _____

Body movements _____

Dress _____

Grooming and hygiene _____

2. Behavior

Level of consciousness _____

Facial expression _____

Speech:

Quality _____

Pace _____

Word choice _____

Mood and affect _____

3. Cognitive Functions
   Orientation:
      Time _____
      Place _____
      Person _____
   Attention span _____
   Recent memory _____
   Remote memory _____
   New learning—Four Unrelated Words Test _____
   Additional testing for aphasia:
      Word comprehension _____
      Reading _____
      Writing _____
      Judgment _____

4. Thought Processes and Perceptions _____
   Thought processes _____
   Thought content _____
   Perceptions _____
   Suicidal thoughts _____

2-1   Regional write-up—mental status examination.

Nursing Diagnoses Commonly Associated with Mental Health Disorders

Impaired **Adjustment**
Anxiety
Acute **Confusion**
Chronic **Confusion**
Ineffective **Coping**
Dysfunctional **Family** processes: Alcoholism
Impaired **Memory**
Disturbed **Personal** identity

Powerlessness
Chronic low **Self-esteem**
Situational low **Self-esteem**
Self-mutilation
Impaired **Social** interaction
Social isolation
Risk for **Suicide**
Risk for **Violence** (self-directed or other-directed)

⇒——— ABNORMAL FINDINGS ———⇐

TABLE 2–1 | Levels of Consciousness

The terms below are commonly used in clinical practice. They spread over a continuum from full alertness to deep coma. The terms are qualitative and therefore are not always reliable. (A quantitative tool that serves the same purpose and eliminates ambiguity is the Glasgow Coma Scale in Chapter 16.) These terms are widely accepted, however, and are useful as long as all co-workers agree on definitions and are consistent in their application.

To increase clarity when using these terms, also record:

1. The level of stimulus used, ranging progressively from
   a. Name called in normal tone of voice
   b. Name called in loud voice
   c. Light touch on person's arm
   d. Vigorous shake of shoulder
   e. Pain applied
2. The person's response
   a. Amount and quality of movement
   b. Presence and coherence of speech
   c. Opens eyes and makes eye contact
3. What the person does on cessation of your stimulus

(1) Alert
Awake or readily aroused, oriented, fully aware of external and internal stimuli, and responds appropriately, conducts meaningful interpersonal interactions

(2) Lethargic (or Somnolent)
Not fully alert, drifts off to sleep when not stimulated, can be aroused to name when called in normal voice but looks drowsy, responds appropriately to questions or commands but thinking seems slow and fuzzy, inattentive, loses train of thought, spontaneous movements are decreased

Adapted from Strub RL, Black FW: *The Mental Status Examination in neurology,* ed 4, Philadelphia, 2000, F.A. Davis.

TABLE 2–1	Levels of Consciousness—cont'd

(3) Obtunded

(Transitional state between lethargy and stupor; some sources omit this level)

Sleeps most of time, difficult to arouse (needs loud shout or vigorous shake), acts confused when aroused, converses in monosyllables, speech may be mumbled and incoherent, requires constant stimulation for even marginal cooperation

(4) Stupor or Semi-Coma

Spontaneously unconscious, responds only to vigorous shake or pain, has appropriate motor response (i.e., withdraws hand to avoid pain), otherwise can only groan, mumble, or move restlessly, but retains reflex activity

(5) Coma

Completely unconscious, makes no response to pain or to any external or internal stimuli (e.g., when suctioned, will not try to push the catheter away). Light coma has some reflex activity but not purposeful movement; deep coma has no motor response

Acute Confusional State (Delirium)

Has clouding of consciousness (dulled cognition, impaired alertness), inattentive, makes incoherent conversation, has impaired recent memory and is confabulatory for recent events, often agitated and has visual hallucinations, disoriented, with confusion worse at night when environmental stimuli are decreased

Chapter Three

Assessment Techniques and the Clinical Setting

ASSESSMENT TECHNIQUES

The skills requisite for the physical examination are inspection, palpation, percussion, and auscultation. The skills are performed one at a time and in this order.

Inspection

Inspection is close careful scrutiny, first of the person as a whole and then of each body system. Inspection begins the moment you first meet the individual and develop a "general survey." (Specific data to consider for the general survey are presented in the following chapter.) As you proceed through the examination, start the assessment of each body system with inspection.

Learn to use each person as his or her own control and compare the right and left sides of the body. The two sides are nearly symmetric. Inspection requires good lighting, adequate exposure, and occasional use of instruments (otoscope, ophthalmoscope, penlight, nasal and vaginal specula) to enlarge your view.

Palpation

Palpation follows and often confirms points you noted during inspection. Palpation applies your sense of touch to assess these factors: texture, temperature, moisture, and organ location and size, as well as any swelling, vibration or pulsation, rigidity or spasticity, crepitation, presence of lumps or masses, and presence of tenderness or pain. Different parts of the hands are best suited for assessing different factors:

- Fingertips—Best for fine tactile discrimination, such as skin texture, swelling, pulsatility, and presence of lumps
- A grasping action of the fingers and thumb—To detect the position, shape, and consistency of an organ or mass
- The dorsa (backs) of hands and fingers—Best for determining temperature because the skin here is thinner than on the palms
- Base of fingers (metacarpophalangeal joints) or ulnar surface of the hand—Vibration

Your palpation technique should be slow and systematic. Warm your hands by kneading them together or holding them under warm water. Identify any tender areas, and palpate them last.

Start with light palpation to detect surface characteristics and accustom the person to being touched.

When deep palpation is needed (as for abdominal contents), intermittent pressure is better than one long, continuous palpation. Avoid any situation in which continuous or deep palpation could cause internal injury or pain.

Bimanual palpation requires the use of both hands to envelop or capture certain body parts or organs, such as the kidneys, uterus, or adnexa, for more precise delimitation.

Percussion

Percussion involves tapping the person's skin with short, sharp strokes to assess underlying structures. The strokes yield a palpable vibration and a characteristic sound that depicts the location, size, and density of the underlying organ.

The Stationary Hand. Hyperextend the middle finger of your nondominant hand (sometimes called the pleximeter) and place its distal portion *firmly* against the person's skin. Avoid the ribs and scapulae. Percussing over a bone yields no data because it always sounds "dull." Lift the rest of the stationary hand up off the person's skin (Fig. 3–1); otherwise, the resting hand will dampen off the produced vibrations, just as a drummer uses the hand to halt a drum roll.

The Striking Hand. Use the middle finger of your dominant hand as the *striking* finger (sometimes called the plexor). Hold your forearm close to the skin surface with your upper arm and shoulder steady but not rigid. The action is all in the wrist, and it *must* be relaxed.

Bounce your middle finger off the stationary one. Aim for just behind the nail bed. Flex the striking finger so that its tip, not the finger pad, makes contact. It hits directly at right angles to the stationary finger.

Percuss two times in this location using even, staccato blows. Lift the striking finger off quickly; a resting finger dampens vibrations. Then move to a new body location and repeat, keeping your technique even (Table 3–1).

TABLE 3–1	Characteristics of Percussion Notes		
	Amplitude	Pitch	Quality
Resonant	Medium loud	Low	Clear, hollow
Hyperresonant	Louder	Lower	Booming
Tympany	Loud	High	Musical and drumlike (like a kettle drum)
Dull	Soft	High	Muffled thud
Flat	Very soft	High	A dead stop of sound; absolute dullness

Auscultation

Auscultation is listening to sounds produced by the body, such as the heart, blood vessels, lungs, and abdomen, through a **stethoscope.**

Choose a stethoscope with two endpieces—a diaphragm and a bell. The **diaphragm** has a flat edge and is best for high-pitched sounds—breath, bowel, and normal heart sounds. Hold the diaphragm firmly against the person's skin, firm enough to leave a slight ring afterward.

The **bell** endpiece has a deep, hollow, cuplike shape. It is best for soft, low-pitched sounds, such as extra heart sounds or murmurs. Hold it lightly against the person's skin, just enough so it forms a perfect seal.

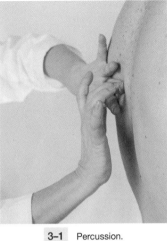

3–1   Percussion.

Duration	Sample Location
Moderate	Over normal lung tissue
Longer	Normal over a child's lung. In an adult, over lungs with abnormal amount of air, such as in emphysema
Sustained longest	Over air-filled viscus (e.g., the stomach, the intestine)
Short	Over relatively dense organs (e.g., liver and spleen)
Very short	When no air is present, or over thigh muscles, bone, or tumor

Pressing harder causes the skin to act as a diaphragm, obliterating the low-pitched sounds.

SETTING

- The examination room should be warm and comfortable, quiet, private, and well lit.
- When possible, stop any distracting noises.
- Discourage interruptions.
- Lighting with natural daylight is best, although artificial light will suffice.
- Position a wall or standing lamp for high intensity lighting.
- The examination table is positioned so that both sides are easily accessible and at a height at which you can stand without stooping.
- The table should be equipped to raise the patient's head up to 45 degrees.
- A roll-up stool is needed for the sections of the examination for which you must be sitting.
- A bedside stand or table should be nearby to allow you to lay out your equipment.

EQUIPMENT

Before the examination, have all your equipment within easy reach and laid out in an organized manner. These items are usually needed for a complete physical examination:

Platform scale with height attachment
Skinfold calipers
Sphygmomanometer
Stethoscope with bell and diaphragm
    endpieces
Thermometer
Flashlight or penlight
Otoscope/ophthalmoscope
Tuning fork
Nasal speculum (if a short, broad speculum is not included with the otoscope)
Tongue depressor
Pocket vision screener
Skin marking pen
Flexible tape measure and ruler marked in centimeters
Reflex hammer
Sharp object (sterile needle or split-tongue blade)
Cotton balls
Bivalve vaginal speculum
Clean gloves
Materials for cytologic study
Lubricant
Fecal occult blood test materials

A SAFER ENVIRONMENT

Designate a "clean" versus a "used" area for handling of your equipment. Distinguish the clean area by one or two disposable paper towels. On the towels, place all the single-use, newly cleaned, or newly alcohol-wiped equipment that you will use on this patient. Equipment that is used frequently on many patients can become a common vehicle for transmission of infection. Use alcohol wipes to clean all equipment that you carry from patient to patient, e.g., your stethoscope endpieces, the reflex hammer, or ruler. As you proceed through the examination, pick up each piece of equipment from the clean area, and, after use on the patient, relegate it to the used area, or throw it directly into the trash.

Take all steps to avoid any possible transmission of infection between patients or between patient and examiner. The single most important step to decrease risk of microorganism transmission is to wash your hands promptly and thoroughly for 10 to 15 seconds (or longer if hands appear visibly soiled). Follow the Centers for Disease Control and Prevention (CDC) guidelines for decreasing transmission of bloodborne and other infections in hospitals (Garner, 1996). These **Standard Precautions** are intended for use with *all* patients regardless of their risk or presumed infection status. They apply to: (1) blood; (2) all body fluids, secretions, and excretions *except sweat,* whether or not they contain visible blood; (3) nonintact skin; and (4) mucous membranes (Table 3–2).

TABLE 3–2	Standard Precautions for Use with All Patients

A. **Wash hands** after touching blood, body fluids, secretions, excretions, and contaminated items. Wash hands immediately after gloves are removed and between patient contacts.

B. **Wear gloves** when touching blood, body fluids, secretions, excretions, items contaminated with these, mucous membranes, and nonintact skin. Change gloves between tasks and procedures on the same patient after contact with material that may contain a high concentration of microorganisms. Remove gloves promptly after use, before touching noncontaminated items, and before going to another patient, and wash hands immediately.

C. **Wear a mask and eye protection** to protect mucous membranes during procedures and patient care activities that are likely to generate splashes of blood, body fluids, secretions, and excretions.

D. **Wear a gown** (clean, nonsterile, appropriate to activity) to protect skin and to prevent soiling of clothing during procedures and patient care activities that are likely to generate splashes of blood, body fluids, secretions, or excretions. Remove a soiled gown promptly and wash hands.

E. **Take care with used patient care equipment** soiled with blood, body fluids, secretions, and excretions; handle it in a manner that prevents skin and mucous membrane exposure, contamination of clothing, and transfer of microorganisms to other patients and environments. Do not use the reusable equipment on another patient until it has been cleaned and reprocessed appropriately. Discard single-use items appropriately.

F. **Design and follow adequate hospital or clinic procedures** for the routine care, cleaning, and disinfection of environmental surfaces, beds, bed rails, bedside equipment, and other frequently touched surfaces.

G. **Take care with used linen** soiled with blood, body fluids, secretions, and excretions; handle, transport, and process this linen in a manner that prevents skin and mucous membrane exposure and contamination of clothing, and that avoids transfer of microorganisms to other patients and environments.

H. **Prevent injuries due to bloodborne pathogens** when using or handling needles, scalpels, and other sharp instruments. Never recap used needles, or manipulate them using body, hands, or direct the point of a needle toward any part of the body; rather, use either a one-handed "scoop" technique or an appropriate mechanical device. Do not remove used needles from disposable syringes by hand, or otherwise bend, break, or manipulate used needles by hand. Place used disposable syringes, needles, scalpel blades, and other sharp items in appropriate puncture-resistant containers.

Use mouthpieces, resuscitation bags, or other ventilation devices instead of mouth-to-mouth resuscitation methods in areas where the need for resuscitation is predictable.

I. **Place in a private room** any patient who contaminates the environment or who does not or cannot assist in appropriate hygiene or environmental control.

Adapted from Garner JS: *Guideline for isolation precautions in hospitals,* Atlanta, 1996, Public Health Service, U.S. Department of Health and Human Services, Centers for Disease Control and Prevention.

APPROACH TO THE CLINICAL SETTING

Preparation for a Complete Assessment

Most people, whether entering the hospital or receiving outpatient care, initially require a complete physical examination. Before you begin, ask the person to empty the bladder and save a urine specimen if needed.

Begin by measuring the person's height, weight, blood pressure, temperature, pulse, and respirations. If needed, measure visual acuity at this time using the Snellen eye chart.

Ask the person to change into an examining gown, leaving the underpants on. Unless your assistance is needed, leave the room as the person undresses.

Consider safety and protect yourself and the patient against the spread of any possible infection. As you reenter the room, wash your hands in the person's presence. This indicates you are protective of the patient and are starting fresh for him or her. Wear gloves when there is potential contact with any body fluids (e.g., mouth or genitalia examination).

Explain each step in the examination and how the person can cooperate. Encourage him or her to ask questions. Keep your own movements slow, methodical, and deliberate.

As you proceed through the examination, avoid distractions and concentrate on one step at a time. The sequence of the steps may differ depending on the age of the patient and your own preference; however, you should establish a system that works for you and stick to it to avoid omissions.

Organize the steps so the person does not change positions too often. Although proper exposure is necessary, use additional drapes to maintain the person's privacy and to prevent chilling.

(See Chapter 20 for the sequence of steps in the complete physical examination.)

The Ill Person

For the ill person in some distress, alter the position during the examination. A patient with shortness of breath or ear pain, for example, may want to sit up, whereas a person with faintness or overwhelming fatigue may want to be supine. Initially, it may be necessary just to examine the body areas appropriate to the problem, collecting a focused or *mini data base.* You may return to finish a complete assessment after the initial distress is resolved.

Episodic or Problem-Centered Assessment

This is for a limited or short-term problem. Here, you collect a focused data base, smaller in scope than the complete assessment. It concerns mainly one problem, one cue complex, or one body system. It is used in all settings—hospital, primary care, or long-term care.

Follow-up Assessment

The status of any identified problems should be evaluated at regular and appropriate intervals. What change has occurred? Is the problem getting better or worse? What coping strategies are used? This type of assessment is used in all settings to follow up short-term or chronic health problems.

For more information on the preparation of infants, children, and older adults for the physical examination, see Jarvis: *Physical Examination and Health Assessment,* 5th ed., pp. 142–145.

Chapter Four

The General Survey, Measurement, Vital Signs, and Pain Assessment

GENERAL SURVEY

The general survey is a study of the whole person, covering the general health state and any obvious physical characteristics. Objective parameters are used to form the general survey, but these apply to the whole person, not just to one body system.

Begin building a general survey from the moment you first encounter the person. What leaves an immediate impression?

As you proceed through the health history, the measurements, and the vital signs, note the following points, which will add up to the general survey: physical appearance, body structure, mobility, and behavior.

PHYSICAL APPEARANCE

Age—The person appears to be his or her stated age.

Sexual development—Development is appropriate for gender and age.

Level of consciousness—The person is alert and oriented, attends to questions, and responds appropriately.

Skin color—Color tone is even, pigmentation varying with genetic background; skin is intact with no obvious lesions.

Facial features—Features are symmetric with movement.

There are no signs of acute distress.

BODY STRUCTURE

Stature—The height appears within normal range for age and genetic heritage.

Nutrition—The weight appears within normal range for height and body build. Body fat distribution is even.

Symmetry—Body parts look equal bilaterally and are in relative proportion to each other.

Posture—The person stands comfortably erect as appropriate for age.

Position—The person sits comfortably in a chair or on the bed or examination table, with arms relaxed at sides and head turned to examiner.

Body build, contour—Proportions are:

1. Arm span (fingertip to fingertip) equals height.
2. Body length from crown to pubis is roughly equal to length from pubis to sole.

Obvious physical deformities—Note any congenital or acquired defects.

MOBILITY

Gait—Normally, the base is as wide as the shoulder width. Foot placement is accurate. The walk is smooth, even, and well balanced; associated movements, such as symmetric arm swing, are present.

Range of motion—Note full mobility for each joint and whether movement is deliberate, accurate, smooth, and coordinated.

No involuntary movement is present.

BEHAVIOR

Facial expression—The person maintains eye contact (unless there is a cultural taboo). Expressions are appropriate to the situation (e.g., thoughtful, serious, or smiling).

Mood and affect—The person is comfortable and cooperative with the examiner and interacts pleasantly.

Speech—Articulation (the ability to form words) is clear and understandable. The stream of speech is fluent, with an even pace. Ideas are conveyed clearly. Word choice is appropriate to culture and education. The person communicates in prevailing language easily by himself or herself or with an interpreter.

Dress—Clothing is appropriate to the climate, looks clean and fits the body, and is appropriate to the person's culture and age group.

Personal hygiene—The person appears clean and groomed appropriately for his or her age, occupation, and socioeconomic group. Hair is groomed or brushed. Woman's make-up is appropriate for age and culture.

MEASUREMENT

WEIGHT

Use a standardized *balance* or *electronic scale.* Instruct the person to remove his or her shoes and heavy outer clothing before standing on the scale. When a sequence of repeated weights is necessary, aim for approximately the same time of day and the same type of clothing worn each time. Record the weight in kilograms and in pounds. Show the person how his or her own weight matches up to the recommended range for height (Table 4–1).

Compare the person's weight with the previous health visit. A recent weight loss may be explained by dieting.

An unexplained weight loss may be a sign of a short-term illness (e.g., fever, infection, disease of the mouth or throat) or a chronic illness (endocrine disease, malignancy, mental health dysfunction).

A weight gain usually reflects overabundant caloric intake, unhealthy eating habits, or a sedentary lifestyle.

Obesity, or the excessive accumulation of fat in the body, is over 120% ideal weight with regard to age, height, and body structure. Obesity occasionally may be due to endocrine disorders, drug therapy (e.g., corticosteroids), or mental depression.

HEIGHT

Use the measuring pole on the balance scale. Align the extended headpiece with the top of the head. The person should be shoeless, standing straight, and looking straight ahead. Heels, buttocks, and shoulders should be in contact with a hard surface.

TABLE 4–1	Height and Weight Tables for Men and Women According to Frame, Ages 25–59		
Height*		**Weight†**	
Feet	Inches	Small Frame	Medium Frame	Large Frame
Men				
5	2	128–134	131–134	138–150
5	3	130–136	133–143	140–153
5	4	132–138	135–145	142–156
5	5	134–140	137–148	144–160
5	6	136–142	139–151	146–164
5	7	138–145	142–154	149–168
5	8	140–148	145–157	152–172
5	9	142–151	148–160	155–176
5	10	144–154	151–163	158–180
5	11	146–157	154–166	161–184
6	0	149–160	157–170	164–188
6	1	152–164	160–174	168–192
6	2	155–168	164–178	172–197
6	3	158–172	167–182	176–202
6	4	162–176	171–187	181–207
Women				
4	10	102–111	109–121	118–131
4	11	103–113	111–123	120–134
5	0	104–115	113–126	122–137
5	1	106–118	115–129	125–140
5	2	108–121	118–132	128–143
5	3	111–124	121–135	131–147
5	4	114–127	124–138	134–151
5	5	117–130	127–141	137–155
5	6	120–133	130–144	140–159
5	7	123–136	133–147	143–163
5	8	126–139	136–150	146–167
5	9	129–142	139–153	149–179
5	10	132–145	142–156	152–173
5	11	135–148	145–159	155–176
6	0	138–151	148–162	158–179

*Shoes with 1-inch heels.
†Weight in pounds. Men: Allow 5 lb of clothing. Women: Allow 3 lb of clothing.

Arm Span or Total Arm Length

Measurement of arm span is useful for situations in which height is difficult to measure, such as in children with cerebral palsy or scoliosis or in aging persons with spinal curvature. Arm span, which is nearly equivalent to height, is sometimes used clinically instead of height.

Ask the person to hold the arms straight out from the sides of the body. Measure the distance from the tip of the middle finger on one hand to that on the other hand.

SKINFOLD THICKNESS

Skinfold thickness measurements provide an estimate of body fat stores or the extent of obesity or undernutrition. The triceps skinfold (TSF) is the site most commonly selected because of its easy accessibility and because standards and techniques are most developed for this site. To measure triceps skinfold thickness:

1. Have the ambulatory person stand with arms hanging freely at the sides and his or her back to the examiner.
2. Using the thumb and forefinger of your left hand, gently grasp a fold of skin and fat on the posterior aspect of the person's upper arm, midway between the acromion process of the scapula and the olecranon process (the tip of the elbow). Gently pull the skinfold away from the underlying muscle.
3. While grasping the skinfold, pick up the calipers with your right hand and depress the spring-loaded lever. Apply caliper jaws horizontally to the fat fold. Release the lever of the calipers while holding the skinfold. Wait 3 seconds, then take a reading. Repeat three times and average the three skinfold measurements (Fig. 4–1).
4. Record measurements to the nearest 5 mm (0.5 cm). Compare the person's measurements with standards by age and sex (see Appendixes H and I on the Evolve website at http://evolve.elsevier.com/Jarvis.

Triceps skinfold values that are 10% below or above standard are suggestive of undernutrition or overnutrition, respectively. Conditions such as edema or subcutaneous emphysema may produce falsely high readings.

♥ DEVELOPMENTAL CARE

Infants and Children

Weight

Weigh an infant on a platform-type balance scale. To check calibration, set the weight at zero and observe the beam balance. Guard the baby so that he or she does not fall. Weigh to the nearest 10 g ($\frac{1}{2}$ oz) for infants and 100 g ($\frac{1}{4}$ lb) for toddlers.

By age 2 or 3 years, use the upright scale. Leave underpants on the child. Some young children are fearful of the rickety standing platform and may prefer sitting on the infant scale. Use the upright scale with preschoolers and school-age children, maintaining modesty with light clothing.

Length

Until age 2 years, measure the infant's body length supine using a horizontal measuring board. Hold the head in the midline. Because the infant normally has flexed legs, extend them momentarily by holding the knees together and pushing them down until the legs are flat on the table. Avoid using a tape measure along the infant's length because this is inaccurate.

By age 2 or 3 years, measure the child's height by standing the child against the pole on the platform scale or against a flat ruler taped to the wall. Encourage the child to stand

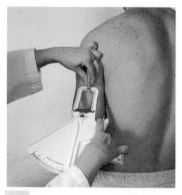

4–1 Measuring triceps skinfold thickness.

straight and tall and to look straight ahead without tilting the head. The shoulders, buttocks, and heels should touch the wall. Hold a book or flat board on the child's head at a right angle to the wall. Mark just under the book or board, noting the measure to the nearest 1 mm ($\frac{1}{8}$ inch).

Head Circumference

Measure the infant's head circumference at birth and at each well child visit up to age 2 years, then yearly up to age 6 years. Circle the tape around the head at the prominent frontal and occipital bones; the widest span is correct. Plot the measurement on standardized growth charts. Compare the infant's head size with that expected for age. A series of measurements is more valuable than a single figure to show the *rate* of head growth.

A newborn's head measures about 32 to 38 cm (average around 34 cm) and is about 2 cm larger than the chest circumference. The chest grows at a faster rate than the cranium; at some time between 6 months and 2 years, both measurements are about the same, and after age 2, the chest circumference is greater than the head circumference.

Measurement of the chest circumference is valuable as a comparison with the head circumference but is not necessarily valuable by itself. Circle the tape around the chest at the nipple line. It should be snug but not so tight as to leave a mark.

The Aging Adult

Weight

An aging person has more prominent bony landmarks than a younger adult. Body weight decreases during the 70s and 80s. This factor is more evident in males, perhaps because of greater muscle shrinkage. The distribution of fat also changes when persons are in their 70s and 80s. Subcutaneous fat is lost from the face and periphery (especially the forearms), and additional fat is deposited in the abdomen and hips.

Height

By their 70s and 80s, many people are shorter than they were in their 60s. This results from shortening of the spinal column due to thinning of the vertebral discs and shortening of the individual vertebrae, as well as postural changes of kyphosis and slight flexion in the knees and hips. Because long bones do not shorten with age, the overall body proportion appears different—a shorter trunk with relatively long extremities.

Kyphosis is an exaggerated posterior curvature of the thoracic spine (humpback). See Table 18–3, p. 468, in Jarvis: *Physical Examination and Health Assessment,* 5th ed.

VITAL SIGNS

TEMPERATURE

The normal oral temperature in a resting person is 37° C (98.6° F), with a range of 35.8° to 37.3° C (96.4° to 99.1° F). The rectal temperature measures 0.4° to 0.5° C (0.7° to 1° F) higher. The normal temperature is influenced by:

- A diurnal cycle of 1° to 1.5° F, with the trough occurring in the early morning hours and the peak occurring in late afternoon to early evening.
- The menstruation cycle in women. Progesterone secretion, occurring with ovulation at midcycle, causes a 0.5° to 1.0° F rise in temperature that continues until menses.
- Exercise. Moderate to hard exercise increases body temperature.
- Age. Wider normal variations occur in infants and young children

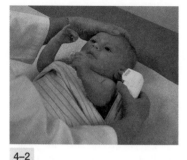

4–2

because of less effective heat control mechanisms. In older adults, temperature is usually lower than in other age groups with a mean of 36.2° C (97.2° F).

The **tympanic membrane thermometer** (TMT) is a noninvasive, nontraumatic device that is rapid and efficient. The probe tip is shaped like an otoscope. Gently place the covered probe tip in the person's ear canal. Do not force it and do not occlude the canal. Activate the device and read the temperature in 2 seconds (Fig. 4–2).

The **electronic thermometer** has the advantages of swift and accurate measurements (usually within 30 seconds) as well as safe, unbreakable, disposable probe covers. The instrument must be fully charged and correctly calibrated. Read the instructions carefully before use. Some types of electronic thermometers use the *same* type of probe cover for oral, rectal, or continuous temperatures, but other manufacturers supply different probes for different routes.

Shake the **glass thermometer**[*] down to 35.5° C (96° F), and place it at the base of the tongue in either of the posterior sublingual pockets, *not* in

front of the tongue. Instruct the person to keep his or her lips closed. Leave in place 3 to 4 minutes if the person is afebrile and up to 8 minutes if febrile. Wait 15 minutes before inserting the thermometer if the person has just taken hot or iced liquids and 2 minutes if he or she has just smoked.

Take a **rectal** temperature only when the other routes are not practical, such as when a tympanic thermometer is not available or for persons who are comatose or confused, in shock, or unable to close the mouth. Wear gloves and insert a lubricated rectal thermometer only 2 to 3 cm (1 inch) into the adult rectum, directed toward the umbilicus. (Note that a glass thermometer will register in 2½ minutes.)

PULSE

Using the pads of your first three fingers, palpate the radial pulse at the flexor aspect of the wrist laterally along the radius bone. Push until you feel the strongest pulsation. If the rhythm is regular, count the number of beats in 30 seconds and multiply by 2. If, however, the rhythm is irregular, count for 1 full minute. As you begin the counting interval, start your count with "zero" for the first pulse felt. The second pulse felt is "one" and so on.

In a resting adult, the normal heart rate range is 60 to 100 beats per minute (bpm), although well-conditioned athletes may have a resting rate as low as 50 bpm. The rate normally varies with age, being more rapid in infancy and childhood and more moderate during adulthood and older years. The rate also varies with gender; after puberty, females have a slightly faster rate than males.

RESPIRATIONS

Normally, a person's breathing is relaxed, regular, automatic, and silent. Most people are unaware of their

---

[*]Note: Due to environmental concerns about possible mercury pollution, and due to concerns about pediatric use, mercury-containing thermometers and sphygmomanometers have been replaced in most medical settings.

breathing, so do not mention that you will be counting the respirations, because sudden awareness may alter the normal pattern. Instead, maintain your position of counting the radial pulse and unobtrusively count the respirations. Count for 30 seconds if respirations are normal or for 1 full minute if you suspect an abnormality. Avoid the 15-second interval because the result can vary by a factor of ±4, which is significant with such a small number.

Respiratory rates are 10 to 20 breaths per minute for adults and are normally more rapid for infants and children. A fairly constant ratio of pulse rate to respiratory rate also exists, which is about 4:1. Normally, both pulse and respiratory rates rise as a response to exercise or anxiety.

BLOOD PRESSURE

Blood pressure is the force of the blood pushing against the side of the vessel wall. The **systolic** pressure is the maximum pressure felt on the artery during left ventricular contraction, or systole. The **diastolic** pressure is the elastic recoil, or resting pressure, that the blood constantly exerts between each contraction. The **pulse pressure** is the difference between the systolic and diastolic pressures and reflects the stroke volume.

The average blood pressure in young adults is 120/80 mm Hg, although this varies normally with many factors, such as:

Age: Normally, there is a gradual rise through childhood and into adult years (Fig. 4–3).
Sex: Before puberty, there is no difference between males and females. After puberty, females usually show a lower blood pressure reading than their male counterparts. After menopause, blood pressure in females is higher than in their male counterparts.

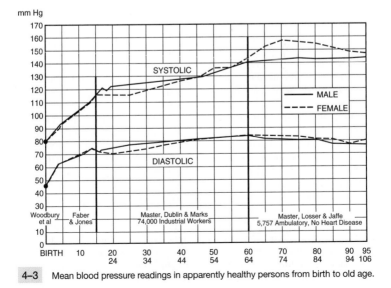

4–3   Mean blood pressure readings in apparently healthy persons from birth to old age.

Race: In the United States, a black adult's blood pressure is usually higher than that of whites of the same age. The incidence of hypertension is twice as high in blacks as in whites. The reasons for this difference are not understood fully but appear to be due to genetic heritage and environmental factors.

Diurnal rhythm: There is a daily cycle of a peak and a trough: Blood pressure climbs to a high in late afternoon or early evening and then declines to an early morning low.

Weight: Blood pressure is higher in obese persons than in persons of normal weight of the same age (including adolescents).

Exercise: Increasing activity yields a proportionate increase in blood pressure. Within 5 minutes of terminating exercise, blood pressure normally returns to baseline.

Emotions: Blood pressure momentarily rises with fear, anger, and pain as a result of stimulation of the sympathetic nervous system.

Stress: Blood pressure is elevated in persons experiencing continual tension because of lifestyle, occupational stress, or life problems.

Blood pressure is measured using a stethoscope and a *sphygmomanometer* of either the mercury or aneroid type.

The cuff consists of an inflatable rubber bladder inside a cloth cover. The width of the rubber bladder should equal 40% of the circumference of the extremity used. The length of the bladder should equal 80% of this circumference.

The size is important; using a cuff that is too narrow yields a falsely high blood pressure. Match the appropriate size cuff to the person's arm size and shape and not to his or her age.

Arm Pressure. A comfortable, relaxed person yields a valid blood pressure. Many people are anxious at the beginning of an examination; allow at least a 5-minute rest before measuring the blood pressure.

The patient may be sitting or lying, with the bare arm supported at the heart level. Palpate the brachial artery, which is located just above the antecubital fossa medially. With the cuff deflated, center it about 2.5 cm (1 inch) above the brachial artery and wrap it evenly.

Now palpate the brachial or the radial artery. Inflate the cuff until the artery pulsation is obliterated and then 20 to 30 mm Hg beyond. This will avoid missing an *auscultatory gap* (i.e., sounds temporarily disappear), which is common with hypertension.

Deflate the cuff quickly and completely, then wait 15 to 30 seconds before reinflating so the blood trapped in the veins can dissipate.

Place the stethoscope over the site of the brachial artery, making a light but airtight seal. (Use the bell endpiece if you have one.) Deflate the cuff slowly and evenly, about 2 mm Hg per heartbeat. Note the points at which you hear the first appearance of sound (the systolic pressure value), the muffling of sound, and the final disappearance of sound. These are phases I, IV, and V of *Korotkoff's sounds.*

In children and adults, phase V (the last audible sound) indicates diastolic pressure. When a variance greater than 10 to 12 mm Hg exists between phases IV and V, however, record *both* phases along with the systolic reading (e.g., 142/98/80). Clear communication is important because results significantly affect diagnosis and planning of care. Table 4–2 presents a list of common errors in blood pressure measurement.

TABLE 4–2	Common Sources of Error in Blood Pressure Measurement

Errors that produce a falsely *high* reading
- Failure to use the appropriate cuff size; a too-narrow cuff gives a higher reading
- Wrapping the cuff too loosely or unevenly; cuff pressure must be exceedingly high to compress the brachial artery
- Recording blood pressure just after a meal, while person is smoking, or while person's bladder is distended
- Failure to have the mercury column vertical
- Deflating the cuff too slowly; this produces venous congestion in the extremity, which falsely elevates diastolic pressure

Errors that produce a falsely *low* reading
- Having the person's arm above the level of the heart (effect of hydrostatic pressure can give an error up to 10 mm Hg in systolic and diastolic pressure)
- Failure to notice an auscultatory gap
- Diminished hearing acuity of the health care professional
- Stethoscope that is too small or too large or has tubing that is too long
- Inability to hear feeble Korotkoff's sounds

Errors that produce *either* falsely *high* or *low* readings
- Inaccurately calibrated manometer
- Defective equipment (e.g., valve, connections)
- Failure to have meniscus of mercury at eye level
- Performing the technique too quickly, with too little attention to details

From Jarvis C: Assessing vital signs. In Bolander VB (Ed): *Sorensen and Luckmann's basic nursing: a pathophysiologic approach,* ed 3, Philadelphia, 1994, W.B. Saunders, p. 620.

If the person is known to have hypertension, is taking antihypertensive medications, or reports a history of fainting or syncope, take the blood pressure reading with him or her in three positions—lying down, sitting, and standing. Normally, a slight decrease (less than 10 mm Hg) in systolic pressure is possible when the position is changed from supine to standing.

Orthostatic hypotension, a drop in systolic pressure of more than 20 mm Hg, may occur with a quick change to a standing position. It is due to abrupt peripheral vasodilation without a compensatory increase in cardiac output. Aging people have the greatest risk of this problem. It also occurs with prolonged bedrest, hypovolemia, and some drugs. Table 4–3 presents further information on hypotension and hypertension.

🌡 DEVELOPMENTAL CARE

The aorta and major arteries tend to harden with age. As the heart pumps against a stiffer aorta, the systolic pressure increases, leading to a widened pulse pressure (see Fig. 4–3 for mean blood pressure readings in apparently healthy persons from birth to old age). With many older people, both the systolic and diastolic pressures increase, making it difficult to distinguish normal aging values from abnormal hypertension.

TABLE 4–3	Abnormalities in Blood Pressure

Hypotension

In normotensive adults:	Below 95/60
In hypertensive adults:	Below the person's average reading, but above 95/60
In children:	Below expected value for age

Occurs With	Rationale
Acute myocardial infarction	Decreased cardiac output
Shock	Decreased cardiac output
Hemorrhage	Decrease in total blood volume
Vasodilation	Decrease in peripheral vascular resistance
Addison's disease (hypofunction of adrenal glands)	

Associated Symptoms and Signs

In conditions of decreased cardiac output, a low blood pressure is accompanied by an increased pulse, dizziness, diaphoresis, confusion, and blurred vision. The skin feels cool and clammy because the superficial blood vessels constrict to shunt blood to the vital organs. An individual having an acute myocardial infarction may also complain of crushing substernal chest pain, high epigastric pain, and shoulder or jaw pain.

Hypertension*

Essential or Primary Hypertension

This occurs from no known cause but is responsible for about 95% of cases of hypertension in adults.

*Hypertension should not be diagnosed by a single measurement. Confirm initial elevated readings on at least two or more readings taken at subsequent visits over one to several weeks (unless severely elevated). When systolic and diastolic pressures fall into different categories, the higher category should be selected to classify the person's blood pressure status.[1]

THE DOPPLER TECHNIQUE

The Doppler technique is used to locate peripheral pulse sites. For blood pressure measurement, the Doppler technique will augment Korotkoff's sounds when they are hard to hear with a stethoscope, such as in critically ill people with a low blood pressure, in infants with small arms, and in obese persons in whom the sounds are muffled by layers of fat. Proper cuff placement is also difficult on an obese person's cone-shaped upper arm. In this situation, you can place the cuff on the more even forearm and hold the Doppler probe over the radial artery (Fig. 4–4). For either location, use this procedure:

- Apply coupling gel to the transducer probe.
- Turn the Doppler probe on.
- Touch the probe to the skin, holding the probe perpendicular to the artery.
- A pulsatile whooshing sound indicates location of the artery. You may need to rotate the probe, but maintain contact with the skin. Do not push the probe too hard or you will wipe out the pulse.

TABLE 4–3	Abnormalities in Blood Pressure—cont'd			
Classification and Follow-up of Blood Pressure for Adults Aged 18 and Older				
Category	Systolic (mm Hg)		Diastolic	Lifestyle Modification
Normal*	<120	and	<80	Encourage
Prehypertension	120–139	or	80–89	Yes‡
Hypertension†				
Stage 1	140–159	or	90–99	Yes, and drug therapy‡
Stage 2	≥160	or	≥100	Yes, and drug therapy‡

Hypertension should not be diagnosed by a single measurement. Confirm initial elevated readings on at least two or more readings taken at subsequent visits over one to several weeks (unless severely elevated). When systolic and diastolic pressures fall into different categories, the higher category should be selected to classify the person's blood pressure status.[1]

*Not taking antihypertensive drugs and not acutely ill. When systolic and diastolic blood pressures fall into different categories, the higher category should be selected to classify the individual's blood pressure status. Isolated systolic hypertension is defined as systolic blood pressure 140 mm Hg or greater and diastolic blood pressure less than 90 mm Hg and staged appropriately. In addition to classifying stages of hypertension on the basis of average blood pressure levels, clinicians should specify presence or absence of target organ disease and additional risk factors. This specificity is important for risk classification and treatment.

†Optimal blood pressure with respect to cardiovascular risk is less than 120/80 mm Hg. However, unusually low readings should be evaluated for clinical significance.

‡Provide advice about lifestyle modifications.

[1]Data from the Seventh Report of the Joint National Committee on Detection, Evaluation and Treatment of High Blood Pressure (JNC-7). Reprinted in *JAMA 289:2560-2572, May 21, 2003.*

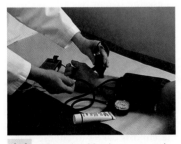

4–4   Measuring blood pressure using the Doppler technique.

- Inflate the cuff until the sounds disappear, then proceed another 20 to 30 mm Hg beyond that point.
- Slowly deflate the cuff, noting the point at which the first whooshing sounds appear. This is the systolic pressure.

- It is difficult to hear the muffling of sound or a reliable disappearance of sounds indicating the diastolic pressure (phases IV and V of Korotkoff's sounds). However, the systolic blood pressure alone gives valuable data on the level of tissue perfusion and on blood flow through patent vessels.

PAIN—THE FIFTH VITAL SIGN

Pain is a highly complex and subjective experience that originates from the central (CNS) or peripheral nervous system (PNS) or both. Pain is defined as "an unpleasant sensory and emotional experience associated with actual or potential tissue damage, or described in terms of such damage. Pain is always subjective" (American

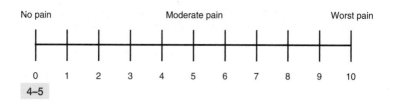

4–5

Pain Society, 1992, p. 250). "Pain is whatever the experiencing person says it is, existing whenever he says it does," (McCaffery, 1968, p. 95). The subjective report is the most reliable indicator of pain. With knowledge that pain occurs on a neurochemical level, the clinician cannot base the diagnosis of pain exclusively on physical exam findings. Physical exam findings can lend support. At this time, x-rays, CAT scans, and MRIs are not sensitive enough to identify minute damage to nerve fibers.

Pain is multidimensional in scope, encompassing physical, affective, and functional domains. Various tools have been developed to capture unidimensional aspects (e.g., intensity) or multidimensional components. Select the pain assessment tool based on its purpose, time involved in administration, and the patient's ability to comprehend and complete the tool.

Pain Rating Scales are unidimensional and are intended to reflect pain intensity. They come in various forms. Pain Rating Scales can indicate a baseline intensity, track changes, and give some degree of evaluation to a treatment modality. **Numeric rating scales** ask the patient to choose a number that rates the level of pain, with 0 indicating no pain and 10 indicating the worst pain. It can be administered verbally or visually along a vertical or horizontal line (Fig. 4–5).

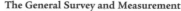 **DEVELOPMENTAL CARE**

Infants

Infants have the same capacity for pain as adults. Preverbal infants are at high risk for undertreatment of pain because of persistent myths and beliefs that infants do not remember pain. Because infants are "preverbal and incapable of self-report," pain assessment is dependent upon behavioral and physiologic clues.

Children 2 years of age can report pain and point to its location. They cannot rate pain intensity at this developmental level. It is helpful to ask the parent or caregiver what words his or her child uses to report pain (e.g., boo-boo, owie). Some children will try to be "grown-up and brave" and often deny having pain in the presence of a stranger or if they are fearful of receiving a "shot." Rating scales can be introduced at 4 or 5 years of age. The Wong-Baker Scale is one example; the child is asked to choose a face that shows "how much hurt you have now." (See *Physical Examination and Health Assessment,* 5th ed., p. 187.) Similarly, the Oucher Scale (Beyer, 1983) has six photographs of young boys' faces with different expressions of pain, ranked on a 0-5 scale of increasing intensity. The child is asked to point at what face best matches his or her hurt/pain.

The Aging Adult

No evidence exists to suggest that older individuals perceive pain to a lesser degree or that sensitivity is diminished. Although pain is a common experience among individuals 65 years of age and older, it is *not* a normal process of aging. Pain indicates pathology/injury. Pain should never be considered something to tolerate or accept in one's later years.

In general, older adults find the numeric scale abstract and have difficulty responding, especially with a fluctuating chronic pain experience. An alternative is the simple **Descriptor Scale** that lists words that describe different levels of pain intensity, such as *no pain, mild pain, moderate pain,* and *severe pain.* Older adults will often respond to scales in which words are selected.

Nursing Diagnoses Commonly Associated with Measurement or Vital Signs Disorders

Adult **Failure** to thrive
Risk for deficient **Fluid** volume
Hyperthermia
Hypothermia
Imbalanced **Nutrition:** less than body requirements
Imbalanced **Nutrition:** more than body requirements

Acute **Pain**
Chronic **Pain**
Bathing/hygiene **Self-care** deficit
Dressing/grooming **Self-care** deficit
Sleep deprivation
Ineffective **Thermoregulation**

Chapter Five

Skin, Hair, and Nails

ANATOMY

The skin has two layers—the outer, highly differentiated **epidermis** and the inner supportive **dermis** (Fig. 5–1). Beneath these layers is a third layer—the insulating **subcutaneous** layer of adipose tissue.

The **sebaceous** glands produce a protective lipid, sebum, which is secreted through the hair follicles. The **eccrine** glands are coiled tubules that open directly onto the skin surface and produce the sweat that helps reduce body temperature. The **apocrine** glands open into hair follicles, become active during puberty, and produce sweat with emotional and sexual stimulation.

The **nails** are hard plates of keratin on the dorsal edges of the fingers and toes (Fig. 5–2). The nail plate is clear, with fine, longitudinal ridges

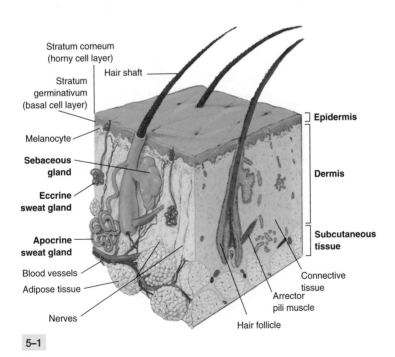

Stratum corneum (horny cell layer)

Stratum germinativum (basal cell layer)

Hair shaft

Melanocyte

Sebaceous gland

Eccrine sweat gland

Apocrine sweat gland

Blood vessels

Adipose tissue

Nerves

Epidermis

Dermis

Subcutaneous tissue

Connective tissue

Arrector pili muscle

Hair follicle

5–1

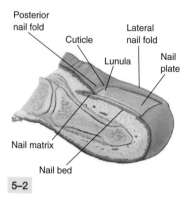

Posterior nail fold
Cuticle
Lunula
Lateral nail fold
Nail plate
Nail matrix
Nail bed

5–2

that become prominent with older age. Nails take their pink color from the underlying nail bed of highly vascular epithelial cells.

CROSS-CULTURAL CARE

Melanin is responsible for the various colors and tones of skin among people from culturally diverse backgrounds. Melanin protects the skin against harmful ultraviolet rays, a genetic advantage accounting for the lower incidence of skin cancer among darkly pigmented black and Native American people.

The hair of black people varies widely in texture. It is very fragile and ranges from long and straight to short, spiraled, thick, and kinky. The hair and scalp have a natural tendency to be dry and require daily combing, gentle brushing, and the application of oil. By comparison, people of Asian backgrounds generally have straight, silky hair.

SUBJECTIVE DATA

1. Previous history of skin disease (allergies, hives, psoriasis, eczema)
2. Change in pigmentation
3. Change in mole (size or color)
4. Excessive dryness or moisture
5. Pruritus
6. Excessive bruising
7. Rash or lesion
8. Medications (any that cause allergic skin response, increased sunlight sensitivity)
9. Hair loss
10. Change in nails
11. Environmental or occupational hazards (sun exposure, toxic chemicals, insect bites)
12. Self-care behaviors (daily hygiene; use of soaps, cosmetics, or chemicals

OBJECTIVE DATA

EQUIPMENT NEEDED
Strong direct lighting (natural daylight is ideal to evaluate skin characteristics but is usually not available in the clinical area)

Small centimeter ruler
Penlight
Gloves

Normal Range of Findings	Abnormal Findings
Inspect and Palpate the Skin	
Color	
General Pigmentation. The skin tone is consistent with genetic background and varies from pinkish tan	

Normal Range of Findings	Abnormal Findings

to ruddy dark tan, or from light to dark brown, and may have yellow or olive overtones. Dark-skinned people normally have areas of lighter pigmentation on the palms, nail beds, and lips.

General pigmentation is darker in sun-exposed areas. Common (benign) pigmentations also occur:

- **Freckles** (ephelides)—a small, flat increase of brown melanin pigment
- **Nevus** (mole)—a proliferation of melanocytes, tan to brown color, flat or raised
- **Birthmarks**—may be tan to brown color

Advise anyone with moles or birthmarks to perform periodic skin self-examinations. Watch for danger signs listed here. Ask a family member to check any areas the person cannot see (e.g., the back).

Widespread Color Change. Note any pallor (white), erythema (red), cyanosis (blue), and jaundice (yellow). In dark-skinned people, the amount of normal pigment may mask color changes. Lips and nail beds may not always be accurate signs. The more reliable sites are those with the least pigmentation, such as under the tongue, the buccal mucosa, the palpebral conjunctiva, and the sclera. Table 5–1 on pp. 47-48 presents specific clues to assessment.

Temperature

Use the backs (dorsa) of your hands and palpate bilaterally. The skin should be warm with equal temperature bilaterally. Hands and feet may be slightly cooler in a cool environment.

Hypothermia. Generalized coolness may be induced, such as in hypothermia used for surgery or high fever. Localized coolness is expected

Danger signs: Abnormal characteristics of pigmented lesions are summarized with the mnemonic **ABCDE:**

Asymmetry of a pigmented lesion.
Border irregularity.
Color variation (areas of black, gray, blue, red, white, pink) or dark black color.
Diameter greater than 6 mm.
Elevation and Enlargement.

Additionally, an individual may report a change in a mole's size, a new pigmented lesion, or the development of itching, burning, or bleeding in a mole. Any of these signs should raise suspicion of malignant melanoma and warrants referral.

General hypothermia accompanies central circulatory disturbance, such as with shock. Localized hypothermia occurs in peripheral arte-

Normal Range of Findings	Abnormal Findings
with an immobilized extremity, as when a limb is in a cast or with an intravenous infusion.	rial insufficiency and in Raynaud's disease because of vasospasm.
Hyperthermia. Generalized hyperthermia occurs with an increased metabolic rate, such as in fever or after heavy exercise. A localized area feels hyperthermic with trauma, infection, or sunburn.	Warm moist skin occurs with hyperthyroidism as a result of hypermetabolic state.

Moisture

Perspiration appears normally on the face, hands, axilla, and skinfolds in response to activity, a warm environment, or anxiety. *Diaphoresis,* or profuse perspiration, accompanies an increased metabolic rate, such as occurs in heavy activity or fever.

Diaphoresis occurs with thyrotoxicosis and with stimulation of the nervous system with anxiety or pain.

Look for dehydration in the oral mucous membranes. Normally, there is none, and the mucous membranes look smooth and moist. Be aware that dark skin may normally look dry and flaky, but this does not necessarily indicate systemic dehydration.

With dehydration, mucous membranes look dry and the lips look parched and cracked. With extreme dryness, the skin is fissured, resembling cracks in a desert.

Texture

Normal skin feels smooth and firm, with an even surface.

Hyperthyroidism—the skin feels smoother and softer, like velvet. Hypothyroidism—the skin feels rough, dry, and flaky.

Thickness

The epidermis is uniformly thin over most of the body, although thickened callus areas are normal on palms and soles. A callus is a circumscribed overgrowth of epidermis and is an adaptation to excessive pressure.

Very thin, shiny skin (atrophic) occurs with arterial insufficiency.

Edema

Edema is fluid accumulating in the intercellular spaces and is not normally present. To check for edema, imprint your thumbs firmly against the ankle malleolus or the tibia. Normally, the skin surface stays smooth when you lift your thumbs. If your pressure leaves a dent in the skin, "pitting" edema is present. Its presence is graded on a

Edema is most evident in dependent parts of the body (feet, ankles, and sacral areas), where the skin looks puffy and tight. Edema makes the hair follicles more prominent, so you note a pigskin or orange-peel look.

Normal Range of Findings	Abnormal Findings

four-point scale: from 1+ for mild edema to 4+ for deep pitting edema. This scale is somewhat subjective; outcomes vary among examiners.

Edema masks normal skin color and obscures pathologic conditions such as jaundice or cyanosis, because the fluid lies between the surface and the pigmented and vascular layers. It makes dark skin look lighter.

Unilateral edema—consider a local or peripheral cause.

Bilateral edema or edema that is generalized over the whole body (anasarca) suggests a central problem such as heart failure or kidney failure.

Mobility and Turgor

Pinch up a large fold of skin on the anterior chest under the clavicle. Mobility is the skin's ease of rising, and turgor is its ability to return to place promptly when released.

Mobility is decreased when edema is present.

Poor turgor is evident in severe dehydration or extreme weight loss; the pinched skin recedes slowly or "tents" and stands by itself.

Vascularity or Bruising

Cherry (senile) angiomas are small, smooth, slightly raised, bright red dots that commonly appear on the trunk in all adults over 30. They normally increase in size and number with aging and are not significant.

Any bruising (ecchymosis) should be consistent with the expected trauma of life. There is normally no venous dilation or varicosity.

Multiple bruises at different stages of healing and excessive bruises above the knees or elbows should raise concern about physical abuse.

Document the presence of any tattoos (a permanent skin design from indelible pigment) on the person's chart. Advise the person that the use of tattoo needles and tattoo parlor equipment of doubtful sterility increases the risk of hepatitis C.

Needle marks or tracks from intravenous injection of street drugs may be visible on the antecubital fossae or forearms or on any available vein.

Lesions

Note:
1. Color
2. Elevation: flat, raised, or pedunculated
3. Pattern or shape: The grouping or distinctness of each lesion, for example, annular, grouped, confluent, linear. The pattern may be characteristic of a certain disease.
4. Size, in centimeters: Use a ruler to measure. Avoid descriptions such as "quarter size" or "pea size."

Lesions are traumatic or pathologic changes in previously normal structures. When a lesion develops on previously unaltered skin, it is **primary.** When a lesion changes over time, however, or changes because of a factor such as scratching or infection, it is **secondary.** Study Table 5–2 for pattern and Tables 5–3 and 5–4, pp. 50–54, for the characteristics of primary and secondary skin lesions.

Normal Range of Findings	Abnormal Findings
5. Location and distribution on body. Is it generalized or localized to area of a specific irritant (around jewelry, watchband, around eyes)? 6. Any exudate? Note its color or odor. Wear a glove if you anticipate contact with blood, mucosa, any body fluid, or an open skin lesion.	
Inspect and Palpate the Hair Color Hair color comes from melanin production and may vary from pale blonde to total black. Graying begins as early as the third decade of life as a result of genetic factors.	
Texture Scalp hair may be fine or thick and may look straight, curly, or kinky. It should look shiny.	Note dull, coarse, or brittle scalp hair.
Lesions The scalp should be clean and free of any lesions or pest inhabitants. Many people normally have seborrhea (dandruff), which is indicated by loose white flakes.	Distinguish dandruff from nits (eggs) of lice, which are oval, adhere to the hair shaft, and cause intense itching.
Inspect and Palpate The Nails Shape and Contour The nail surface is normally slightly curved or flat, and the posterior and lateral nail folds are smooth and rounded. Nail edges are smooth, rounded, and clean, suggesting adequate self-care.	Spoon nails (concave curves) may occur with iron-deficiency anemia. Paronychia (inflammation of base of nail) occurs with trauma or infection. Jagged nails, nails bitten to the quick, or traumatized nail folds from chronic nervous picking suggest nervous habits. Chronically dirty nails suggest poor self-care or occupations in which it is impossible to keep them clean.
View the index finger at its profile and note the angle of the nail base; it should be about 160 degrees. The nail	Clubbing of nails occurs with congenital, chronic, cyanotic heart disease and with emphysema and

Normal Range of Findings	Abnormal Findings
base is firm to palpation. Curved nails with a convex profile are a variation of normal. They may look like clubbed nails, but notice that the angle between nail base and nail is normal (i.e., 160 degrees or less).	chronic bronchitis. In early clubbing, the angle straightens out to 180 degrees and the nail base feels spongy to palpation (see Fig. 12–9, p. XXX in Jarvis: *Physical Examination and Health Assessment,* 5th ed.).

Consistency

The nail surface is smooth and regular, not brittle or splitting.

Pits, transverse grooves, or lines may indicate a nutrient deficiency or may accompany acute illness with disturbed nail growth.

Nail thickness is uniform.

Nails thickened, ridged, with arterial insufficiency.

The nail is firmly adherent to the nail bed, and the nail base is firm to palpation.

A spongy nail base accompanies clubbing.

Color

The translucent nail plate shows a pink nail bed underneath.

Cyanosis or marked pallor.

Dark-skinned people may have brown-black pigmented areas or linear bands or streaks along the nail edge. Many people normally have white hairline linear markings from trauma or picking at the cuticle. Note any abnormal markings in the nail beds.

Brown linear streaks are abnormal in light-skinned people and may indicate melanoma.

Splinter hemorrhages occur with subacute bacterial endocarditis; transverse ridges, or Beau's lines, occur with trauma.

Capillary Refill. Depress the nail edge to blanch and then release, noting the return of color. Normally, color return is instant or within a few seconds in a cold environment. This indicates the status of the peripheral circulation. A sluggish color return takes longer than 1 or 2 seconds.

Cyanotic nail beds or sluggish color return—consider cardiovascular or respiratory dysfunction.

DEVELOPMENTAL CARE

Infants

General Pigmentation. Black newborns initially have lighter-toned skin than their parents. Their full melanotic color is evident in the nail beds and scrotal folds.

The **Mongolian spot** is a common variation of hyperpigmentation in black, Native American, Hispanic, and

Bruising is a common soft tissue injury that follows a rapid, traumatic, or breech birth.

Normal Range of Findings	Abnormal Findings

Asian newborns as a result of deep dermal melanocytes. It is a blue-black to purple macular area usually found at the sacrum or buttocks. It gradually fades during the first year of life.

Multiple bruises in various stages of healing, or pattern injury, which do not match history, suggest physical abuse.

Adolescents

The increase in sebaceous gland activity creates increased oiliness and acne.

The Pregnant Female

Striae are jagged linear "stretch marks" of silver to pink that appear during the second trimester on the abdomen, breasts, and sometimes on the thighs. They occur in one-half of all pregnancies and fade after delivery but do not disappear. On the abdomen, the **linea nigra** appears as a brownish black line down the midline.

Chloasma is an irregular brown patch of hyperpigmentation on the face. It may occur with pregnancy or in women taking oral contraceptive pills. Chloasma disappears after delivery or cessation of pill use.

Vascular spiders occur in two-thirds of pregnancies in white women but less often in black women. These lesions have tiny red centers with radiating branches and occur on the face, neck, upper chest, and arms.

The Aging Adult

Skin Color and Pigmentation. Senile lentigines are commonly called liver spots and are small, flat, brown macules that appear after extensive sun exposure on the forearms and dorsa of the hands. They are not malignant and require no treatment.

Moisture. Dry skin (xerosis) is common. The skin itches and appears flaky and loose.

Texture. Acrochordons, or "skin tags," are overgrowths of normal skin that form a stalk and occur frequently on the eyelids, cheeks, neck, axillae, and trunk.

Normal Range of Findings	Abnormal Findings

Thickness. With aging, the skin looks as thin as parchment and subcutaneous fat diminishes. Thinner skin is evident over the dorsae of the hands, forearms, lower legs, feet, and bony prominences.

Mobility and Turgor. Turgor is decreased (less elasticity), and the skin recedes slowly or "tents" and stands by itself.

Hair. Hair growth decreases, and the amount decreases in the axillae and pubic areas. After menopause, white women may develop bristly hairs on the chin or upper lip, as a result of unopposed androgens.

In men, coarse terminal hairs develop in the ears, nose, and eyebrows, although the beard is unchanged. Male pattern balding, or **alopecia,** is a genetic trait. It is usually a gradual receding of the anterior hairline in a symmetric W shape.

In men and women, scalp hair gradually turns gray because of a decrease in melanocyte function.

Nails. Nail growth rate decreases, and local injuries in the nail matrix may produce longitudinal ridges. The surface may be brittle or peeling and sometimes is yellowed. Toenails also are thickened and may grow misshapen, almost grotesque. The thickening can be a process of aging or is due to chronic peripheral vascular disease.

For more information on assessment of skin, hair, and nails, see Jarvis: *Physical Examination and Health Assessment,* 5th ed., pp. 221–270.

Fungal infections are common in aging, with thickened, crumbling toenails and erythematous scaling on contiguous skin surfaces.

TEACH SKIN SELF-EXAMINATION

Teach all adults to examine their skin once a month, using the ABCDE rule to raise warning signals of any suspicious lesions. Use a well-lit room that has a full-length mirror. It helps to have a small handheld mirror. Ask a relative

Normal Range of Findings	Abnormal Findings

to search skin areas difficult to see (e.g., behind ears, back of neck, back). Follow the sequence outlined below and report any suspicious lesions promptly to a physician or nurse.

1. Undress completely. Check forearms, palms, space between fingers. Turn over hands and study the backs.
2. Face mirror, bend arms at elbows. Study arms in mirror.
3. Face mirror and study entire body front. Start at face and neck, working over torso and down to lower legs.
4. Pivot to have right side facing mirror. Study sides of upper arms, working down to ankles. Repeat with left side.
5. With back to mirror, study buttocks, thighs, lower legs.
6. Use handheld mirror to study upper back.
7. Use handheld mirror to study scalp, lifting the hair. A blow-dryer on a cool setting helps to lift hair.
8. Sit on chair or bed. Study insides of each leg and soles of feet. Use small mirror to help.

Summary Checklist

For a PDA-downloadable version go to http://evolve.elsevier.com/Jarvis.

1. **Inspect the skin:**
   Color
   General pigmentation
   Areas of hypopigmentation or hyperpigmentation
   Abnormal color changes
2. **Palpate the skin:**
   Temperature
   Moisture
   Texture
   Thickness
   Edema
   Mobility and turgor
   Vascularity or bruising

3. **Note any lesions:**
   Color
   Shape and configuration
   Size
   Location and distribution on body
4. **Inspect and palpate the hair:**
   Texture
   Distribution
   Any scalp lesions
5. **Inspect and palpate the nails:**
   Shape and contour
   Consistency
   Color
6. **Teach skin self-examination**

Nursing Diagnoses Commonly Associated
with Skin, Hair, and Nail Disorders

Disturbed **Body** image
Deficient **Fluid** volume
Risk for **Infection**
Deficient **Knowledge**
Pain
Self-care deficit: bathing/hygiene

Chronic low **Self-esteem**
Self-mutilation
Impaired **Skin** integrity
Ineffective **Thermoregulation**
Impaired **Tissue** integrity
Risk for **Trauma**

ABNORMAL FINDINGS

TABLE 5–1	Detecting Color Changes in Light and Dark Skin	
Etiology	Light Skin	Dark Skin
Pallor		
Anemia—decreased hematocrit Shock—decreased perfusion, vasoconstriction	Generalized pallor	Brown skin appears yellow-brown, dull; black skin appears ashen gray, dull; skin loses its healthy glow Check areas with least pigmentation, such as conjunctivae, mucous membranes
Local arterial insufficiency	Marked localized pallor, e.g., lower extremities, especially when elevated	Ashen gray, dull; cool to palpation
Albinism—total absence of pigment melanin throughout the integument	Whitish pink	Tan, cream, white
Vitiligo—patchy depigmentation from destruction of melanocytes	Patchy milky white spots, often symmetric bilaterally	Same
Cyanosis		
Increased amount of unoxygenated hemoglobin Central—chronic heart and lung disease cause arterial desaturation Peripheral—exposure to cold, anxiety	Dusky blue Nail beds dusky	Dark but dull, lifeless Only severe cyanosis is apparent in skin—check conjunctivae, oral mucosa, nail beds

Continued

TABLE 5–1	Detecting Color Changes in Light and Dark Skin—cont'd	
Etiology	Light Skin	Dark Skin
Erythema		
Hyperemia—increased blood flow through engorged arterioles, such as in inflammation, fever, alcohol intake, blushing	Red, bright pink	Purplish tinge, but difficult to see; palpate for increased warmth with inflammation, for taut skin, and for hardening of deep tissues
Polycythemia—increased red blood cells, capillary stasis	Ruddy blue in face, oral mucosa, conjunctivae, hands and feet	Well-concealed by pigment Check for redness in lips.
Carbon monoxide poisoning	Bright cherry red in face and upper torso	Cherry red color in nail beds, lips, and oral mucosa
Venous stasis—decreased blood flow from area, engorged venules	Dusky rubor of dependent extremities; a prelude to necrosis with pressure sores	Easily masked; use palpation for warmth of edema
Jaundice		
Increased serum bilirubin, over 2 to 3 mg/100 ml, due to liver inflammation or hemolytic disease such as after severe burns or some infections	Yellow in sclerae, hard palate, mucous membranes, then over skin	Check sclera for yellow near limbus; do not mistake normal yellowish fatty deposits in the periphery under the eyelids for jaundice Jaundice best noted in junction of hard and soft palate and also in palms
Carotenemia—increased serum carotene from ingestion of large amounts of carotene-rich foods	Yellow-orange in forehead, palms and soles, and nasolabial folds, but no yellowing in sclerae or mucous membranes	Yellow-orange tinge in palms and soles
Uremia—renal failure causes retained urochrome pigments in the blood	Orange-green or gray overlying pallor of anemia; may also have ecchymoses and purpura	Easily masked by dark skin; rely on laboratory and clinical findings

TABLE 5-1	Detecting Color Changes in Light and Dark Skin—cont'd	
Etiology	Light Skin	Dark Skin
Brown-Tan		
Addison's disease—cortisol deficiency stimulates increased melanin production	Bronzed appearance, an "eternal tan," most apparent around nipples, perineum, genitalia, and pressure points (inner thighs, buttocks, elbows, axillae)	Easily masked by dark skin; rely on laboratory and clinical findings
Café-au-lait spots—due to increased melanin pigment in basal cell layer	Tan to light brown, irregularly shaped, oval patches with well-defined borders	

TABLE 5–2 | Common Shapes of Skin Lesions

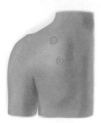

ANNULAR: circular lesions that begin in center and spread to periphery (e.g., ringworm, tinea versicolor, pityriasis rosea)

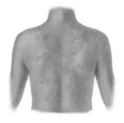

CONFLUENT: lesions that run together (e.g., urticaria)

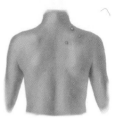

DISCRETE: distinct, individual lesions that remain separate

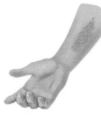

GROUPED: clusters of lesions (e.g., vesicles of contact dermatitis)

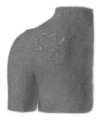

GYRATE: twisted, coiled spiral, or snakelike lesions

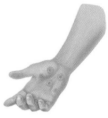

IRIS or **TARGET:** lesions that resemble iris of eye, concentric rings of lesions

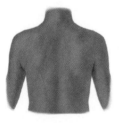

LINEAR: lesions take form of a scratch, streak, line, or stripe

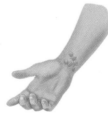

POLYCYCLIC: annular lesions that grow together

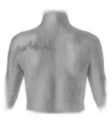

ZOSTERIFORM: lesions take a linear arrangement along a nerve route (e.g., herpes zoster)

TABLE 5–3	Primary Skin Lesions*

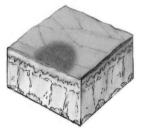

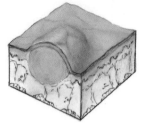

MACULE: Solely a color change, flat and circumscribed, less than 1 cm. Examples: freckle, flat nevus, hypopigmentation, petechia, measles, scarlet fever
PATCH: Macule larger than 1 cm. Examples: Mongolian spot, vitiligo, café-au-lait spot, chloasma, measles rash

PAPULE: Something you can palpate, i.e., solid, elevated, circumscribed lesion less than 1 cm in diameter. Examples: elevated nevus (mole), lichen planus, molluscum, wart (verruca)
PLAQUE: Papules coalesce wider than 1 cm to form a plateaulike, disc-shaped lesion. Examples: psoriasis, lichen planus

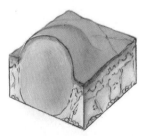

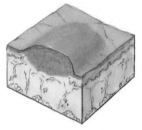

NODULE: Solid, elevated, hard or soft lesion larger than 1 cm; may extend deeper into dermis than papule. Examples: xanthoma, fibroma, intradermal nevus
TUMOR: Lesion larger than a few centimeters in diameter, firm or soft, deeper into dermis; may be benign or malignant. Examples: lipoma, hemangioma

WHEAL: Superficial, raised, transient, and erythematous lesion; has a slightly irregular shape due to edema (fluid held diffusely in the tissues). Examples: mosquito bite, allergic reaction, dermographism
URTICARIA (HIVES): Wheals coalesce to form extensive reaction, intensely pruritic.

*The immediate result of a specific causative factor; primary lesions develop on previously unaltered skin.

Continued

TABLE 5–3	Primary Skin Lesions—cont'd

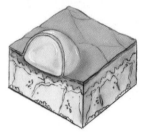

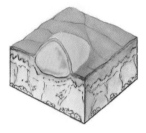

VESICLE: Elevated cavity containing free clear fluid, up to 1 cm. Examples: herpes simplex, early varicella (chickenpox), herpes zoster (shingles), contact dermatitis

BULLA: Larger than 1 cm in diameter; usually single chambered (unilocular); superficial in epidermis; it is thin walled, so it ruptures easily. Examples: friction blister, pemphigus, burns, contact dermatitis

PUSTULE: Turbid fluid (pus) in the cavity; circumscribed and elevated. Examples: impetigo, acne

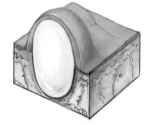

CYST: Encapsulated, fluid-filled ➤ cavity in dermis or subcutaneous layer that tensely elevates skin. Examples: sebaceous cyst, wen

TABLE 5–4 | Secondary Skin Lesions*

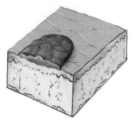

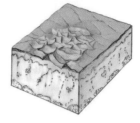

CRUST: Thickened, dried-out exudate left when vesicles or pustules burst or dry up. Color can be red-brown, honey, or yellow, depending on the fluid's ingredients (blood, serum, pus). Examples: impetigo (dry, honey colored), weeping eczematous dermatitis, scab following abrasion

SCALE: Compact, desiccated flakes of skin, dry or greasy, silvery or white, from shedding of dead excess keratin cells. Examples: following drug reaction (laminated sheets), psoriasis (silver, micalike) seborrheic dermatitis (yellow, greasy), eczema, (large, adherent, laminated), dry skin

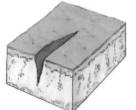

◀ **FISSURE:** Linear crack with abrupt edges, extending into dermis, dry or moist. Examples: cheilosis at corners of mouth due to excess moisture; athlete's foot

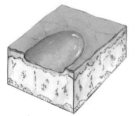

◀ **EROSION:** Scooped-out but shallow depression. Superficial lesion, epidermis is lost, and the lesion is moist but there is no bleeding. Heals without scar because erosion does not extend into dermis.

---

*Resulting from a change in a primary lesion due to the passage of time; an evolutionary change.
Note: Combinations of primary and secondary lesions may coexist in the same person. Such combined designations may be termed *papulosquamous, maculopapular, vesiculopustular,* or *papulovesicular.*

Continued

TABLE 5–4 | Secondary Skin Lesions—cont'd

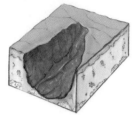

ULCER: Deeper depression, extending into dermis, irregularly shaped. It may bleed and leaves scar when heals. Examples: stasis ulcer, pressure sore, chancre

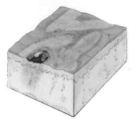

EXCORIATION: Self-inflicted abrasion; superficial and sometimes crusted. Examples: scratches from intense itching from insect bite, scabies, dermatitis, varicella

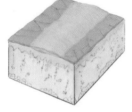

SCAR: After a skin lesion is repaired, normal tissue is lost and replaced with connective tissue (collagen). This is a permanent fibrotic change. Examples: healed area of surgery or injury, acne

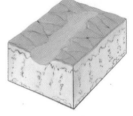

ATROPHIC SCAR: Resulting skin level depressed with loss of tissue; a thinning of the epidermis. Examples: striae

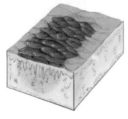

LICHENIFICATION: Prolonged intense scratching eventually thickens the skin and produces tightly packed sets of papules: looks like surface of moss (or lichen).

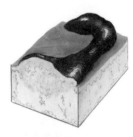

KELOID: Hypertrophic scar. The resulting skin level is elevated by excess scar tissue, which is invasive beyond the site of original injury. May increase long after healing occurs; looks smooth, rubbery, "clawlike." Higher incidence among blacks.

Chapter Six

Head, Face, and Neck, Including Regional Lymphatics

ANATOMY

The head and neck have a rich supply of lymph nodes (Fig. 6–1). The nodes are small oval clusters of lymphatic tissue. They filter the lymph and engulf pathogens, thereby preventing potentially harmful substances from entering the circulation.

The neck contains many structures lying in close proximity (Fig. 6–2). The major neck muscles are the **sternomastoid** and the **trapezius** on the upper back. The carotid artery and internal jugular vein lie beneath the sternomastoid muscle. (Assessment of the neck vessels is discussed in Chapter 12.) The **thyroid gland** straddles the trachea, and its two lobes each curve posteriorly between the trachea and sternomastoid muscle.

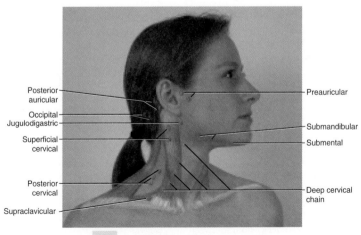

Posterior auricular
Occipital
Jugulodigastric
Superficial cervical
Posterior cervical
Supraclavicular

Preauricular
Submandibular
Submental
Deep cervical chain

6–1 Lymph nodes of the head and neck.

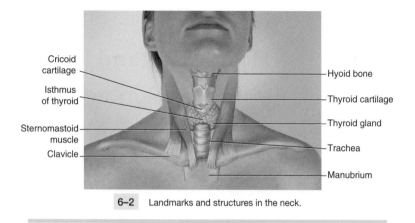

6–2   Landmarks and structures in the neck.

1. Headache
2. Head injury
3. Dizziness

4. Neck pain
5. Limitation of motion
6. Lumps or swelling

Normal Range of Findings	Abnormal Findings
The Head	
Inspect and Palpate the Skull	
Normocephalic describes a round, symmetric skull appropriately related to body size.	Microcephaly—abnormally small head.
	Macrocephaly—abnormally large head (e.g., hydrocephaly and acromegaly). (See Table 13–1, p. 292 in Jarvis: *Physical Examination and Health Assessment,* 5th ed.)
The skull normally feels symmetric and smooth. The cranial bones with normal protrusions are the forehead, the lateral edge of each parietal bone, the occipital bone, and the mastoid process behind each ear. There is no tenderness to palpation.	Lumps, depressions, or abnormal protrusions.
Palpate the temporal artery above the zygomatic (cheek) bone between the eye and top of the ear.	
Palpate the temporomandibular joints located anterior to each ear as	

Normal Range of Findings	Abnormal Findings
the person opens the mouth, and note normally smooth movement with no limitation or tenderness.	Crepitation, limited range of motion, or tenderness.

Inspect the Face

Note the facial expression and its appropriateness to behavior or reported mood. Anxiety is common in hospitalized or ill persons.

Note symmetry of eyebrows, palpebral fissures, nasolabial folds, and sides of the mouth. Note any abnormal facial structures (coarse facial features, exophthalmos, changes in skin color or pigmentation), or any abnormal swelling. Also note any involuntary movements (tics) in the facial muscles. Normally, there are none.

Hostility or embarrassment. Tense, rigid muscles may indicate anxiety or pain; a flat affect may indicate depression.

Marked asymmetry may be seen with central brain lesion (e.g., CVA) or with peripheral cranial nerve VII damage (e.g., Bell's palsy). (See Table 13–4, p. 296, in Jarvis: *Physical Examination and Health Assessment,* 5th ed.)

Edema in the face is noted first around the eyes (periorbital) and the cheeks, where the subcutaneous tissue is relatively loose.

Note grinding of jaws, tics or fasciculations, or excessive blinking.

The Neck
Inspect and Palpate the Neck

Symmetry. Head position is in the midline; accessory neck muscles are symmetric.

Head tilt occurs with muscle spasm.
Head and neck rigidity occurs with arthritis.

Range of Motion. Ask the person to touch the chin to the chest, turn the head to the right and left, try to touch each ear to the shoulder (without elevating shoulders), and extend the head backward. When the neck is supple, motion is smooth and controlled.

Note any limitation of movement.
Note pain at any particular movement.
Note ratchety movement or limitation of movement, which may be due to cervical arthritis or inflammation of neck muscles. With arthritis, the neck is rigid and the person turns at the shoulders rather than the neck.

Lymph Nodes. Using a gentle circular motion of your finger pads and beginning with the preauricular lymph nodes in front of the ear, palpate the 10 groups of lymph nodes in a routine order. Be systematic and thorough. Use gentle pressure because strong pressure could push the nodes into the neck muscles. It is usually most efficient to palpate with both

Lymphadenopathy is disease of the lymph nodes with enlargement to >1 cm from infection, allergy, or neoplasm.

The following are commonly associated with lymphadenopathy but are not definitive in all circumstances:
• Acute infection—nodes are bilateral, enlarged, warm, tender, and firm but freely movable.

Normal Range of Findings	Abnormal Findings

hands, comparing the two sides for the symmetry.

If any nodes are palpable, note their location, size, shape, delimitation (discrete or matted together), mobility, consistency, and tenderness. Cervical nodes often are palpable in healthy persons, although palpability decreases with age. Normal nodes feel movable, discrete, soft, and nontender.

If nodes are enlarged or tender, check the area they drain for the source of the problem. Look proximal (upstream) to the location of the node; for example, those nodes in the upper cervical or submandibular area often relate to inflammation or a neoplasm in the head and neck. Follow up on or refer your findings. An enlarged lymph node deserves prompt attention, particularly when you cannot find the source of the problem.

Thyroid Gland. Position a standing lamp to shine tangentially across the neck to highlight any possible swelling. Supply the person with a glass of water, and first inspect the neck as the person takes a sip and swallows. Thyroid tissue moves up with a swallow.

To palpate the thyroid, move behind the person (Fig. 6–3). Ask him

- Chronic inflammation—e.g., in tuberculosis the nodes are clumped.
- Cancerous nodes are hard, unilateral, nontender, and fixed.
- Nodes in persons with HIV infection are enlarged, firm, nontender, and mobile. Occipital lymphadenopathy is common.
- A single, enlarged, nontender, hard left supraclavicular node may indicate a neoplasm in the thorax or abdomen.
- Painless, rubbery, discrete nodes that appear gradually occur with Hodgkin's lymphoma.

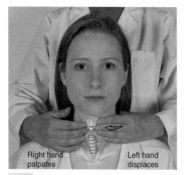

Right hand palpates   Left hand displaces

6–3

Normal Range of Findings	Abnormal Findings

or her to sit up very straight and then to bend the head slightly forward and to the right. This will relax the neck muscles. Use the fingers of your left hand to push the trachea slightly to the right.

Curve your right fingers between the trachea and the sternomastoid muscle, retracting it slightly, and ask the person to take a sip of water. The thyroid moves up under your fingers with the trachea and larynx as the person swallows. Reverse the procedure for the left side.

Usually you cannot palpate a normal adult thyroid. If the person has a long, thin neck, you some-times can feel the thyroid isthmus over the tracheal rings. The lateral lobes usually are not palpable; check them for enlargement, consistency, symmetry, and the presence of nodules.

Abnormalities include enlarged lobes that are easily palpated before swallowing or that are tender to palpation, or the presence of nodules or lumps (see Table 13–2, p. 293, in Jarvis: *Physical Examination and Health Assessment,* 5th ed.).

DEVELOPMENTAL CARE

Infants and Children. An infant's head size is measured with measuring tape at each visit up to age 2. (Measurement of head circumference is presented in detail in Chapter 4.)

Gently palpate the skull and fontanels while the infant is calm and in a somewhat sitting position (crying, lying down, or vomiting may cause the anterior fontanel to look full and bulging). The skull should feel smooth and fused except at the fontanels. The fontanels feel firm, slightly concave, and well defined against the edges of the cranial bones.

You may see slight arterial pulsations in the anterior fontanel.

The posterior fontanel may not be palpable at birth. If it is, it measures 1 cm and closes by age 1 to 2 months. The anterior fontanel may be small at

Microcephaly—Head circumference below norms for age.

Macrocephaly—Head that is enlarged for age or rapidly increasing in size. This may be due to hydrocephalus (increased cerebrospinal fluid).

A true tense or bulging fontanel occurs with acute increased intracranial pressure.

Depressed and sunken fontanels occur with dehydration or malnutrition.

Marked pulsations occur with increased intracranial pressure.

Delayed closure or larger than normal fontanels occur with hydrocephalus, Down syndrome, hypothyroidism, or rickets.

Normal Range of Findings	Abnormal Findings
birth and enlarge to 2.5 cm by 2.5 cm. A large diameter of 4 to 5 cm occasionally may be normal under 6 months.	A small fontanel is a sign of microcephaly, as is early closure.
The anterior fontanel closes between 9 months and 2 years. Early closure may be insignificant if head growth proceeds normally.	
During infancy, cervical lymph nodes are not normally palpable, but a child's lymph nodes are: They feel more prominent than an adult's until puberty when lymphoid tissue begins to atrophy. Palpable nodes less than 3 mm are normal. They may be up to 1 cm in size in the cervical and inguinal areas but are discrete, move easily, and are nontender. Children have a higher incidence of infection, so you will expect a greater incidence of inflammatory adenopathy. There should be no other mass in the neck .	Cervical nodes larger than 1 cm are considered enlarged. Thyroglossal duct cyst—cystic lymph node high up in the midline, that is freely movable and that rises up during swallowing. Supraclavicular nodes enlarge with Hodgkin's disease.
The Pregnant Female. The thyroid gland may be normally palpable during pregnancy as a result of hyperplasia of the tissue and increased vascularity.	
The Aging Adult. In some aging adults, a mild rhythmic tremor of the head is normal. *Senile tremors* are benign and include head nodding (as if saying yes or no) and tongue protrusion.	
If some teeth have been lost, the lower face looks unusually small, with the mouth sunken in.	
The neck may show an increased cervical concave curve when the head and jaw are extended forward to compensate for kyphosis of the spine. During the examination, direct the aging person to perform range of motion slowly; he or she may experience dizziness with side movements.	
For more information on assessment of the head and neck, see Jarvis: *Physical Examination and Health Assessment,* 5th ed., pp. 271–279.	

Summary Checklist

For a PDA-downloadable version go to http://evolve.elsevier.com/Jarvis.

1. Inspect and palpate the skull:
General size and contour
Note any deformities, lumps, tenderness
Palpate temporal artery and temporomandibular joint

2. Inspect the face:
Facial expression
Symmetry of movement (cranial nerve VII)
Any involuntary movements, edema, lesions

3. Inspect and palpate the neck:
Active range of motion
Enlargement of lymph nodes or thyroid gland

Nursing Diagnoses Commonly Associated with Head and Neck Disorders

Risk for ineffective **Airway** clearance
Disturbed **Body** image
Risk for deficient **Fluid** volume
Risk for **Infection**

Pain
Impaired **Physical** mobility
Disturbed **Sensory** perception
Impaired **Swallowing**

Chapter Seven

Eyes

The eye is the sensory organ of vision. The eyelids protect the eye from injury, strong light, and dust (Fig. 7–1). The **palpebral fissure** is the open space between the eyelids.

The exposed part of the eye has a transparent protective covering, the **conjunctiva.** The *palpebral* conjunctiva lines the lids and is clear, with many small blood vessels. It forms a deep recess and then folds back over the eye. The *bulbar* conjunctiva overlays the eyeball, with the white sclera showing through. At the limbus, the conjunctiva merges with the cornea. The **cornea** covers and protects the iris and pupil.

The eye is a sphere composed of three concentric coats: (1) the outer fibrous **sclera,** (2) the middle vascular **choroid,** and (3) the inner nervous **retina** (Fig. 7–2). Inside the retina is the transparent vitreous body.

The retina is the visual receptive layer of the eye in which light waves are changed into nerve impulses. The **ocular fundus** is the area of retina visible through the ophthalmoscope (Fig. 7–3).

The **optic disc** is the area in which fibers from the retina converge to form the optic nerve. The **macula** is the area of sharpest vision.

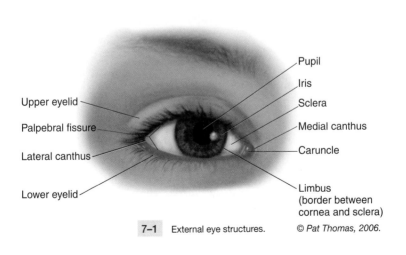

Upper eyelid

Palpebral fissure

Lateral canthus

Lower eyelid

Pupil

Iris

Sclera

Medial canthus

Caruncle

Limbus
(border between
cornea and sclera)

7–1   External eye structures.   © *Pat Thomas, 2006.*

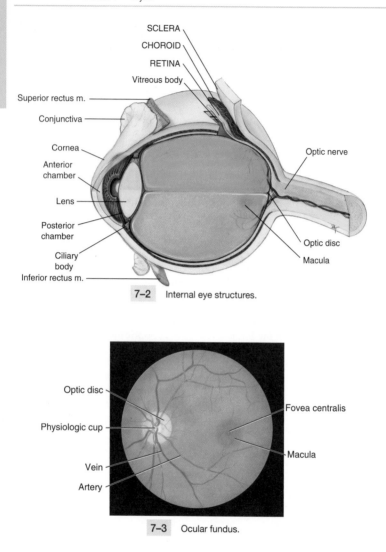

7-2   Internal eye structures.

7-3   Ocular fundus.

CROSS-CULTURAL CARE

Racial differences are evident in the palpebral fissures. Persons of Asian origin are often identified by their characteristic eyes, whereas the presence of narrowed palpebral fissures in non-Asian individuals may be diagnostic of a serious congenital anomaly, *Down syndrome.*

Individuals with darker irides have darker retinas behind them. Individuals with light retinas generally have better night vision but can suffer discomfort in an environment that has too much light.

SUBJECTIVE DATA

1. Vision difficulty (decreased acuity, blurring, blind spots)
2. Pain
3. Strabismus, diplopia
4. Redness, swelling
5. Watering, discharge
6. Past history of ocular problems
7. Glaucoma
8. Use of glasses or contact lenses
9. Self-care behaviors (vision last tested, method of care for contacts or glasses, efforts to protect eyes)

OBJECTIVE DATA

EQUIPMENT NEEDED
Snellen eye chart
Handheld visual screener
Opaque card or occluder
Penlight
Ophthalmoscope

Normal Range of Findings	Abnormal Findings
Test Central Visual Acuity **Snellen Eye Chart** Position the person on a mark exactly 20 feet from the chart. If the person wears glasses or contact lenses, leave them on. Shield one eye at a time during the test. Ask the person to read through the chart to the smallest line of letters possible.	Hesitancy, squinting, leaning forward, misreading letters.
Record the result using the numeric fraction at the end of the last successful line read. Indicate whether any letters were missed and whether corrective lenses were worn, e.g., "O.D.* 20/30—1, with glasses."	
Normal visual acuity is 20/20. The top number (numerator) indicates the distance the person is standing from the chart; the denominator gives the distance at which a normal eye can read a particular line.	The larger the denominator, the poorer the vision. If vision is poorer than 20/30, refer to an ophthalmologist or optometrist. Impaired vision may be due to refractive error, opacity in the media (cornea, lens, vitreous), or disorder in the retina or optic pathway.
Near Vision For people over 40 years of age or for those who report increasing difficulty reading, test near vision using a handheld vision screener with various sizes	

*O.D., oculus dexter, or right eye.

Normal Range of Findings	Abnormal Findings

of print (e.g., a Jaeger card). Hold the card in good light about 35 cm (14 inches) from the eye. Test each eye separately with glasses on. A normal result is "14/14" in each eye, read without hesitancy and without moving the card closer or farther away.

Presbyopia, the decrease in power of accommodation with aging, is suggested when the person moves the card farther away.

Test Visual Fields
Confrontation Test

Position yourself at eye level with the patient and about 2 feet away. Direct him or her to cover one eye with an opaque card and to look straight at you with the other eye. Hold a pencil or your finger as a target midline between you and the other person and slowly advance it in from the periphery in several directions (upward, downward, temporally, nasally).

Ask the person to say "now" as the object is first seen; this should be just as you see the object also.

If the person is unable to see the object as you do, the test suggests peripheral field loss. Refer the person for more precise testing using a tangent screen.

Inspect Extraocular Muscle Function
Diagnostic Positions Test

Leading the eyes through the six *cardinal positions of gaze* will elicit any muscle weakness during movement. Ask the person to hold the head steady and follow the movement of your finger, pen, or penlight only with the eyes. Hold the target object back about 12 inches so the person can focus on it comfortably; move it to each of the six positions, hold it momentarily, then move it back to center. Progress clockwise (Fig. 7–4). A normal response is parallel tracking of the object with both eyes.

In addition to parallel movement, note any **nystagmus,** a fine oscillating movement best seen around the iris. Mild nystagmus at extreme lateral gaze is normal; nystagmus at any other position is not.

Eye movement is not parallel. Failure to follow in a certain direction indicates weakness of an extraocular muscle (EOM) or dysfunction of the cranial nerve that innervates it.

Nystagmus occurs with disease of the semicircular canals in the ears, a paretic eye muscle, multiple sclerosis, or brain lesion.

Normal Range of Findings	Abnormal Findings

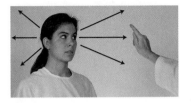

7–4

Finally, note that the upper eyelid continues to overlap the superior part of the iris, even during downward movement.

A white rim of sclera between the lid and the iris, referred to as "lid lag," occurs with hyperthyroidism.

Inspect External Ocular Structures

General

Note the person's ability to move around the room with vision functioning well enough to avoid obstacles and respond to your directions. The facial expression is relaxed with adequate vision.

Groping with hands.

Squinting or craning forward.

Eyebrows

Normally, the eyebrows are present bilaterally, move symmetrically as the facial expression changes, and have no scaling or lesions.

Absent lateral third of eyebrows with hypothyroidism.
Unequal or absent movement with nerve damage.
Scaling with seborrhea.

Eyelids and Lashes

The upper lids normally overlap the superior part of the iris and approximate completely when closed. The skin is intact without redness, swelling, discharge, or lesions.

The palpebral fissures are horizontal in non-Asians, whereas palpebral fissures of Asians normally have an upward slant.

The eyelashes are evenly distributed along the lid margins and curve outward.

Lid lag occurs with hyperthyroidism.
Incomplete closure creates risk for corneal damage.
Ptosis—drooping of upper lid.

Periorbital edema, lesions.

Ectropion and entropion (Table 7–2, p. 76).

Normal Range of Findings	Abnormal Findings

Eyeballs

The eyeballs are aligned normally with no protrusion or sunken appearance. Blacks may normally have a slight protrusion of the eyeball beyond the supraorbital ridge.

Exophthalmos—protruding eyes (see Table 7–2).
Enophthalmos—sunken eyes.

Conjunctiva and Sclera

Ask the person to look up. Using your thumbs, slide the lower lids down along the bony orbital rim. Take care not to push against the eyeball. Inspect the exposed area. The eyeball looks moist and glossy. Numerous small blood vessels normally show through the transparent conjunctiva. Otherwise, the conjunctivae are clear and show the normal color of the structure below—pink over the lower lids and white over the sclera. Note any color change, swelling, or lesions.

General reddening (see Table 7–2).
Cyanosis of the lower lids.
Pallor near the outer canthus of the lower lid may indicate anemia (the inner canthus normally contains less pigment).

The sclera is china white, although blacks occasionally have a gray-blue or "muddy" color to the sclera. Dark-skinned people may have small brown macules (like freckles) on the sclera; do not confuse these with foreign bodies or petechiae. Blacks may have yellowish fatty deposits beneath the lids away from the cornea. Do not confuse these yellow spots with the overall scleral yellowing that accompanies jaundice.

Scleral icterus is a yellowing of the sclera extending up to the cornea, indicating jaundice.
Tenderness, foreign body, discharge, or lesions.

Inspect Anterior Eyeball Structures

Cornea and Lens

Shine a light from the side across the cornea and check for smoothness and clarity. There should be no opacities (cloudiness) in the cornea, in the anterior chamber, or in the lens behind the pupil. Do not confuse **arcus senilis** with an opacity. This is a normal finding in aging persons and is described on page 74.

A corneal abrasion causes irregular ridges in reflected light, usually visible only with fluorescein stain.

Normal Range of Findings	Abnormal Findings

Iris and Pupils

The iris normally has a round regular shape and an even coloration. Normally, the pupils appear round, regular, and of equal size in both eyes. In adults, resting size is from 3 to 5 mm. A small number of people (5%) have pupils of two different sizes, a condition called **anisocoria.**

Irregular shape.

To test the **pupillary light reflex,** darken the room and ask the person to gaze into the distance. (This dilates the pupils.) Advance a light in from the side,* and note the response. Normally, you will see (1) constriction of the same-sided pupil (a *direct light reflex*) and (2) simultaneous constriction of the other pupil (a *consensual light reflex*).

Unequally sized pupils call for consideration of a central nervous system injury.
Dilated pupils.
Dilated and fixed pupils.
Constricted pupils.
Unequal or no response to light (Table 7–3, p. 78).

Test for **accommodation** by asking the person to focus on a distant object. This process dilates the pupils. Then have the person shift the gaze to a near object, such as your finger held about 7 to 8 cm (3 inches) from the nose. A normal response includes (1) pupillary constriction and (2) convergence of the axes of the eyes.

Absence of constriction or convergence.
Asymmetric response.

Record the normal response to these maneuvers as PERRLA, or *Pupils Equal, Round, React to Light,* and *Accommodation.*

Inspect the Ocular Fundus

Darken the room to help dilate the pupils. Remove eyeglasses from yourself or the other person; they obstruct close movement, and you can com-

---

*Always advance the light in from the *side* to test the light reflex. If you advance from the front, the pupils will constrict to accommodate for near vision. Thus, you do not know what the pure response to the light would have been.

Normal Range of Findings	Abnormal Findings

pensate for their correction by using the diopter setting. Contact lenses can be left in.

Select the large round aperture with the white light for routine examination. If the pupils are small, use the smaller white light.

Tell the person, "Please keep looking at that light switch [or mark] on the wall across the room, even though my head will get in the way." Staring at a distant, fixed object helps dilate the pupils and hold the retinal structures still.

Match sides with the person: that is, hold the ophthalmoscope in your *right* hand up to your *right* eye to view the person's *right* eye (Fig. 7–5). You must do this to avoid bumping noses during the procedure. Place your free hand on the person's shoulder or forehead.

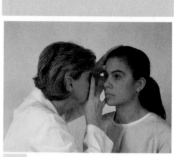

7–5

Systematically inspect the structures in the ocular fundus: (1) optic disc, (2) retinal vessels, (3) general background, and (4) macula (see Fig. 7–3). (Note that the illustration shows a large area of the fundus. Your actual view through the ophthalmoscope is much smaller, slightly larger than 1 disc diameter.)

Optic Disc

The most prominent landmark is the optic disc, located on the nasal side of the retina. Explore these characteristics:

1. Color—Creamy yellow-orange to pink
2. Shape—Round or oval
3. Margins—Distinct, sharply demarcated, though the nasal edge may be slightly fuzzy
4. Cup-disc ratio—Distinctness varies. When visible, cup is a brighter yellow-white than rest of the disc. Its width is not more than one-half the disc diameter.

Pallor. Hyperemia.

Irregular.
Blurred margins.

Cup extending to the disc border (see Table 14–9, p. 340, in Jarvis: *Physical Examination and Health Assessment,* 5th ed.).

Normal Range of Findings	Abnormal Findings

Retinal Vessels

Follow a paired artery and vein out to the periphery in the four quadrants (see Fig. 7–3), noting these points:

1. Number—A paired artery and vein pass to each quadrant. Vessels look straighter at the nasal side.

2. Color—Arteries are brighter red than veins. They also have the arterial light reflex, a thin stripe of light down the middle.

3. A:V ratio—The ratio comparing the artery-to-vein width is 2:3 or 4:5.

4. Caliber—Arteries and veins show a regular decrease in caliber as they extend to periphery.

5. AV (arteriovenous) crossing—An artery and vein may cross paths. This is not significant if within 2 disc diameters (DD) of disc and if no sign of interruption in blood flow. There should be no indenting or displacing of vessel.

6. Tortuosity—Mild vessel twisting when present in both eyes is usually congenital and not significant.

7. Pulsations—Present in veins near the disc as their drainage meets the intermittent pressure of arterial systole. (Often hard to see.)

Abnormal findings:

Absence of major vessels.

Arteries too constricted. Veins dilated.

Focal constriction. Neovascularization.

Crossings more than 2 DD away from disc.
Nicking or pinching of underlying vessel.
Vessel engorged peripheral to crossing.

Extreme tortuosity or marked asymmetry in two eyes.

Absent pulsations (see Table 14–9, p. 340 in Jarvis: *Physical Examination and Health Assessment,* 5th ed.).

General Background of the Fundus

The color normally varies from light red to dark brown-red, generally corresponding with the person's skin color. There should be no lesions obstructing the retinal structures.

Abnormal lesions—hemorrhages, exudates, microaneurysms.

Macula

The macula is 1 DD in size and is located 2 DD temporal to the disc. Inspect this area last in the funduscopic examination. A bright light on this area of central vision causes some watering, discomfort, and pupillary constriction. Note that the normal

Normal Range of Findings	Abnormal Findings
color of the area is somewhat darker than the rest of the fundus but even and homogeneous. Clumped pigment may occur with aging.	Clumped pigment occurs with trauma or retinal detachment. Hemorrhage or exudate in the macula occurs with senile macular degeneration.

♦ DEVELOPMENTAL CARE

Infants and Children. With a newborn, test **light perception** using the blink reflex; neonates blink in response to bright light. The pupillary light reflex also shows that the pupils constrict in response to light.

Testing for **strabismus** (squint, crossed eye) is an important screening measure during early childhood. Untreated strabismus can lead to permanent visual damage, called **amblyopia ex anopsia.** Early recognition and treatment are essential.

Check the **corneal light reflex** by shining a light toward the child's eyes. The light should be reflected at exactly the same spot in the two corneas. Some asymmetry (where one light falls off center) under age 6 months is normal.

Many infants have an **epicanthal fold,** an excess skinfold extending over the inner corner of the eye, partly or totally overlapping the inner canthus. This occurs frequently in Asian children and in 20% of whites. In non-Asians, it disappears as the child grows, usually by age 10 years. While they are present, epicanthal folds give a false appearance of malalignment, called **pseudostrabismus,** but the corneal light reflex is normal.

Asian infants normally have an upward slant of the palpebral fissures. Entropion, a turning inward of the eyelid, is normally found in some Asian children. If the lashes do not abrade the cornea, it is not significant.

Abnormal Findings (continued):

Absent blinking.
Absent pupillary light reflex, especially after 3 weeks, indicates blindness.

Diagnosis after age 6 years has a poor prognosis.

Asymmetry in the corneal light reflex after 6 months is abnormal, and the infant must be referred.

An upward lateral slope together with epicanthal folds and hypertelorism (large spacing between the eyes) occurs with Down syndrome.

Normal Range of Findings	Abnormal Findings

The Aging Adult

The eyebrows may show a loss of the outer one-third to one-half of hair. The remaining brow hair is coarse. Because of atrophy of elastic tissue, the skin around the eyes may show wrinkles or crow's feet. The upper lid may be so elongated as to rest on the lashes (Table 7–1 on p. 74).

The eyes may appear sunken because of atrophy of the orbital fat. The orbital fat may also herniate, causing bulging at the lower lids and inner third of the upper lids.

Atrophy of the levator palpebrae muscle causes a partial ptosis. In contrast with the baggy lids previously described, ptosis is an actual drooping.

The lower lid may drop away from the globe, **ectropion.** Then tears cannot drain into the out-turned puncta. Alternately, **entropion,** or a turning inward of the lower lid, may irritate the eye from friction of lashes (see Table 7–2 on p. 76).

Tear production may decrease, causing the eyes to look dry and lusterless and the person to report a burning sensation. **Pingueculae** commonly show on the sclera (see Table 7–1). These yellowish elevated nodules are due to a thickening of the bulbar conjunctiva from prolonged exposure to sun, wind, and dust. Pingueculae appear at the 3- and 9-o'clock positions, first on the nasal side, then on the temporal side.

Distinguish pingueculae from the abnormal **pterygium,** an opacity also on the bulbar conjunctiva but that grows over the cornea and may block vision.

The cornea may look cloudy with age. **Arcus senilis** is commonly seen around the cornea (see Table 7–1). This is a gray-white arc or circle around the limbus due to deposition of lipid material. As more lipid accumulates, the cornea may look thickened and raised, but the arcus has no effect on vision.

Xanthelasma are soft, raised, yellow plaques occurring on the lids of the inner canthus (see Table 7–1). These commonly occur around the fifth decade of life and more frequently in women. Xanthelasma oc-

TABLE 7–1 | Aging Eye Changes

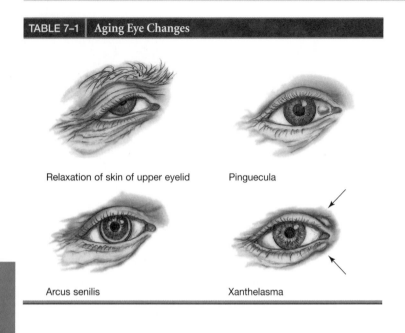

Relaxation of skin of upper eyelid

Pinguecula

Arcus senilis

Xanthelasma

Normal Range of Findings	Abnormal Findings
cur with both high and normal blood levels of cholesterol and have no pathologic significance. Pupils are small, and the pupillary light reflex may be slowed. The lens loses transparency and appears opaque. In the ocular fundus, the blood vessels appear pale, narrow, and attenuated. Arterioles appear pale and straight, with a narrow light reflex. More AV crossing defects occur. A normal development on the retinal surface are **drusen,** or benign degenerative hyaline deposits. They are small, round, yellow dots that are scattered haphazardly on the retina. Although they do not occur in a pattern, drusen are usually symmetrically placed in the two eyes. They have no effect on vision.	Drusen are easily confused with the abnormal finding of *hard exudates* (see Table 14–10, p. 341, in Jarvis: *Physical Examination and Health Assessment,* 5th ed.).

Summary Checklist

For a PDA-downloadable version go to http://evolve.elsevier.com/Jarvis.

1. **Test visual acuity:**
   Snellen eye chart
   Near vision (those older than
      40 years or those having diffi-
      culty reading)
2. **Test visual fields:**
   Confrontation test
3. **Inspect extraocular muscle
   (EOM) function:**
   Corneal light reflex
   Diagnostic positions test
4. **Inspect external eye structures:**
   General
   Eyebrows
   Eyelids and lashes
   Eyeball alignment
   Conjunctivae and sclerae

5. **Inspect anterior eyeball
   structures:**
   Cornea and lens
   Iris and pupil
      Size, shape, and equality
      Pupillary light reflex
      Accommodation
6. **Inspect the ocular fundus:**
   Optic disc (color, shape, margins,
      cup/disc ratio)
   Retinal vessels (number, color,
      artery/vein [A/V] ratio, caliber,
      arteriovenous [AV] crossings,
      tortuosity, pulsations)
   General background (color,
      integrity)
   Macula

Nursing Diagnoses Commonly Associated with the Eyes and Visual Disorders

Activity intolerance
Anxiety
Impaired **Home** maintenance

Pain
Self-care deficit
Disturbed visual **Sensory** perception

ABNORMAL FINDINGS

TABLE 7–2	Abnormalities in the Eyelids

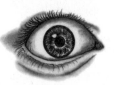

Exophthalmos (Protruding Eyes)

Exophthalmos is a forward displacement associated with thyroid disease. Note "lid lag": The upper lid rests well above the limbus, and white sclera is visible.

Ptosis (Drooping Upper Lid)

Ptosis occurs from neuromuscular weakness (e.g., myasthenia gravis), oculomotor cranial nerve III damage, or sympathetic nerve damage (e.g., Horner's syndrome).

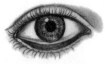

Ectropion

The lower lid is loose and rolling out, and does not approximate to eyeball. Puncta cannot siphon tears effectively, so excess tearing results. Exposed palpebral conjunctiva increases risk for inflammation.

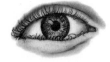

Entropion

The lower lid rolls in as a result of spasm of lids or contraction of scar tissue. Lashes may irritate cornea.

TABLE 7–2 | Abnormalities in the Eyelids

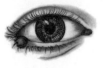

Hordeolum (Stye)

Hordeolum is a localized staphylococcal infection of the hair follicles at the lid margin. It is painful, red, and swollen, and resembles a pustule at the lid margin.

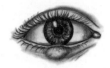

Chalazion

A beady nodule protruding on the lid, chalazion is an infection or retention cyst of a meibomian gland. It is a nontender, firm, discrete swelling with freely movable skin overlying the nodule. If it becomes inflamed, it points inside and not on the lid margin (in contrast with a stye).

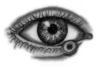

Basal Cell Carcinoma

Carcinoma is rare, but it occurs most often on the lower lid. It looks like a papule with an ulcerated center. The edges are rolled out and pearly.

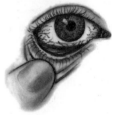

Conjunctivitis

Infection of the conjunctiva shows red, beefy-looking vessels at periphery but looks clearer around iris. This is common due to bacterial or viral infection, allergy, or chemical irritant. Often accompanies an upper respiratory infection. Purulent discharge accompanies bacterial infection.

TABLE 7–3	Abnormalities in the Pupil

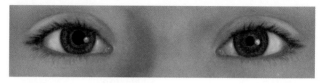

Unequal Pupil Size—Anisocoria

Although anisocoria exists normally in 5% of the population, a person with this may have central nervous system disease.

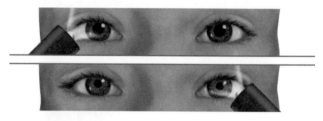

Monocular Blindness

When light is directed to the blind eye, there is no response. When light is directed to the normal eye, both pupils constrict (direct and consensual response to light) as long as the oculomotor nerve is intact.

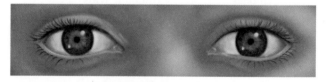

Constricted and Fixed Pupils—Miosis

Miosis occurs with the use of pilocarpine drops for glaucoma treatment, the use of narcotics, with iritis, and with brain damage of the pons.

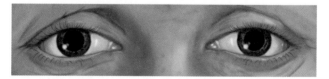

Dilated and Fixed Pupils—Mydriasis

Enlarged pupils occur with stimulation of the sympathic nervous system, reaction of sympathomimetic drugs, use of dilating drops, acute glaucoma, and past or recent trauma. Enlarged pupils may also indicate central nervous system injury, circulatory arrest, or deep anesthesia.

The ear is the sensory organ for hearing and maintaining equilibrium. The external ear is the **auricle,** or **pinna,** and consists of movable cartilage and skin (Fig. 8–1).

The external ear funnels sound into its opening, the **external auditory canal.** The canal is a cul-de-sac 2.5 to 3 cm long in the adult and has a slight S-curve (Fig. 8–2).

The middle ear is a tiny, air-filled cavity inside the temporal bone containing the tiny auditory ossicles: the *malleus, incus,* and *stapes.*

The inner ear contains the *bony labyrinth,* which holds the sensory organs for equilibrium and hearing.

The **tympanic membrane,** or **eardrum,** separates the external and middle ear (Fig. 8–3). It is translucent, with a pearly gray color and a prominent cone of light in the anteroinferior quadrant, which is the reflection of the otoscope light.

The parts of the malleus show through the translucent drum; these are the *umbo,* the *manubrium,* and the *short process.*

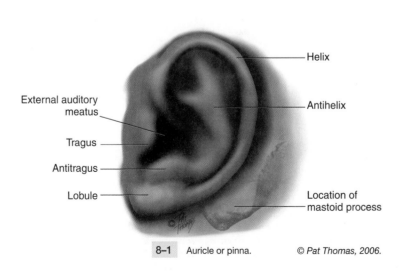

8–1   Auricle or pinna.   © Pat Thomas, 2006.

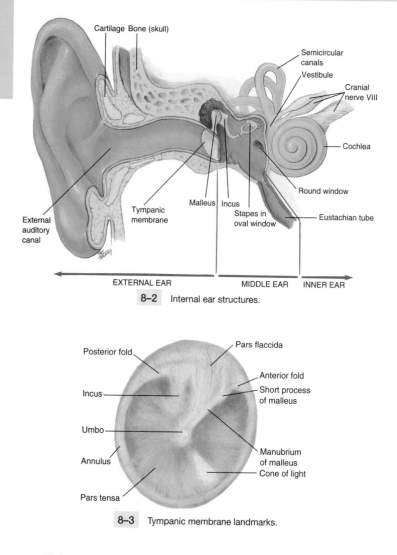

8-2   Internal ear structures.

8-3   Tympanic membrane landmarks.

CROSS-CULTURAL CARE

Cerumen is genetically determined and comes in two major types: (1) Dry cerumen, which is gray, flaky, and frequently forms a thin mass in the ear canal, and (2) wet cerumen, which is honey to dark brown and moist. Asians and Native Americans have an 84% frequency of dry cerumen, whereas blacks have a 99% occurrence and whites a 97% frequency of wet cerumen (Overfield, 1995).

Middle ear infection (otitis media) is one of the most common illnesses in children. The incidence and severity are increased in Native Americans, Alaskans, Canadian Inuits, and Hispanics (Terris, Magit, and Davidson, 1995).

SUBJECTIVE DATA

1. Earaches
2. Infections
3. Discharge
4. Hearing loss
5. Environmental noise
6. Tinnitus
7. Vertigo
8. Self-care behaviors (hearing last checked, method of cleaning ears)

OBJECTIVE DATA

PREPARATION
Position the adult sitting up straight with his or her head at your eye level.

EQUIPMENT NEEDED
Otoscope with bright light (fresh batteries give off white, not yellow, light)
Pneumatic bulb attachment, sometimes used with infant or young child
Tuning forks in 512 and 1024 Hz

Normal Range of Findings	Abnormal Findings
Inspect and Palpate the External Ear	
Size and Shape	
The ears are of equal size bilaterally with no swelling or thickening.	*Microtia*—Ears smaller than 4 cm vertically. *Macrotia*—Ears larger than 10 cm vertically. Edema.
Skin Condition	
The skin is intact, with no lumps or lesions. *Darwin's tubercle,* a small painless nodule at the helix, is sometimes present. This is a congenital variation and is not significant.	Reddened, excessively warm skin indicates inflammation. Crusts and scaling occur with otitis externa and with eczema, contact dermatitis, and seborrhea. Enlarged tender lymph nodes in the region indicate inflammation of the pinna or mastoid process. Tophi, sebaceous crust, chondrodermatitis, keloid, carcinoma (see Table 15–2, p. 364, in Jarvis: *Physical Examination and Health Assessment,* 5th ed.)
Tenderness	
The pinna and the tragus should feel firm, and movement should produce no pain. Palpating the mastoid process should be painless.	Pain with movement occurs with otitis externa and furuncle. Pain at the mastoid process may indicate mastoiditis or lymphadenitis of the posterior auricular node.

Normal Range of Findings	Abnormal Findings

External Auditory Meatus

There should be no swelling, redness, or discharge.

Atresia—Absence or closure of the ear canal.

A sticky yellow discharge accompanies otitis externa, or it may indicate otitis media if the drum has ruptured.

Some cerumen is usually present. The color varies from gray-yellow to light brown and black, and the texture varies from moist and waxy to dry and desiccated.

Impacted cerumen is a common cause of conductive hearing loss.

The Otoscopic Examination

Choose the largest speculum that will fit comfortably. Tilt the person's head slightly away from you toward the opposite shoulder. This method brings the obliquely sloping eardrum into better view.

Pull the pinna up and back on an adult or older child (Fig. 8–4); this helps straighten the S-shape of the canal. (Pull the pinna down on an infant or child under 3 years of age.)

Hold the otoscope upside down along your fingers and have the dorsum (back) of your hand along the person's cheek braced to steady the otoscope (see Fig. 8–4).

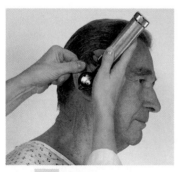

8–4   Using an otoscope.

Normal Range of Findings	Abnormal Findings

External Canal

Note any redness and swelling, lesions, foreign bodies, or discharge. If any discharge is present, note the color and odor. (Also clean any discharge off the speculum before examining the other ear to avoid contamination with possibly infectious material.) For a person with a hearing aid, note any irritation on the canal wall from poorly fitting ear molds.

Redness and swelling occur with otitis externa; the canal may be completely closed with swelling.

Purulent otorrhea suggests otitis externa or suggests otitis media if the drum has ruptured.

Frank blood or clear watery drainage (cerebrospinal fluid leak) after trauma suggests basal skull fracture and warrants immediate referral. Cerebrospinal fluid feels oily and tests positive for glucose.

Foreign body, exostosis, polyp, furuncle (see Table 15–3, p. 366, in Jarvis: *Physical Examination and Health Assessment,* 5th ed.).

Tympanic Membrane

Color and Characteristics. The normal eardrum is shiny and translucent, with a pearl-gray color (see Fig. 8–3). The cone-shaped light reflex is prominent in the anterior inferior quadrant (at the 5-o'clock position in the right drum and the 7-o'clock position in the left drum). This is the reflection of the otoscope light. Sections of the malleus are visible through the translucent drum—the umbo, manubrium, and short process. (Infrequently, the incus behind the drum shows as a whitish haze in the upper posterior area.) At the periphery, the annulus looks whiter and denser.

Position. The eardrum is flat, slightly pulled in at the center, and flutters when the person performs the Valsalva maneuver or holds the nose and swallows (insufflation). These maneuvers assess drum mobility. Avoid them with an aging person, because they may disrupt equilibrium. Also avoid middle ear insufflation in a person with an upper respiratory tract infection, because it could propel infectious matter into the middle ear.

Yellow-amber color of the drum occurs with serous otitis media.

Red color occurs with acute otitis media.

Absent or distorted landmarks.

Air/fluid level or air bubbles behind the drum indicate serous otitis media (Table 8–1, p. 88).

Retracted drum due to vacuum in middle ear.

Bulging drum from increased pressure.

Eardrum does not move (see Table 8–1).

Normal Range of Findings	Abnormal Findings
Integrity of Membrane. The normal tympanic membrane is intact. Some adults may show scarring or a dense white patch on the drum as a sequela of repeated ear infections.	Perforation shows as a dark oval area or as a larger opening on the drum (see Table 8–1). Vesicles on drum.

Test Hearing Acuity

Whispered Voice Test

Test one ear at a time while masking hearing in the other ear by placing one finger on the tragus and rapidly pushing it in and out of the auditory meatus. Shield your lips. With your head 30 to 60 cm (1 to 2 feet) from the person's ear, exhale and whisper slowly some two-syllable words, such as "Tuesday," "armchair," "baseball," and "fourteen." Normally, the person repeats each word correctly after you say it.

The person is unable to hear whispered words. A whisper is a high-frequency sound and is used to detect high-tone loss.

Tuning Fork Tests

Tuning fork tests measure hearing by air conduction (AC) or bone conduction (BC) in which the sound vibrates through the cranial bones to the inner ear. The AC route through the ear canal and middle ear is usually the more sensitive route.

The **Weber test** is valuable when a person reports hearing better with one ear than the other. Place a vibrating tuning fork in the midline of the person's skull and ask if the tone sounds the same in both ears or better in one. The person should hear the tone by bone conduction through the skull, and it should sound equally loud in both ears.

Sound lateralizes to one ear when there is a hearing loss (see Table 15–6, pp. 371 and 372, in Jarvis: *Physical Examination and Health Assessment,* 5th ed.).

The **Rinne test** compares AC and BC sound. Place the stem of the vibrating tuning fork on the person's mastoid process and ask him or her to signal when the sound goes away. Quickly invert the fork so the vibrating end is near the ear canal: the person should still hear a sound. Normally, the sound is heard twice as

Normal Range of Findings	Abnormal Findings

long by AC (next to the ear canal) as by BC (through the mastoid process). A normal response is a positive Rinne test, or "AC > BC." Repeat with the other ear.

Ratio of AC to BC is altered with hearing loss.

Sound is heard longer by bone conduction with a conductive loss.

DEVELOPMENTAL CARE

Infants and Young Children

The top of the pinna should match an imaginary line extending from the corner of the eye to the occiput, and the ear should be positioned within 10 degrees of vertical.

Low-set ears or deviation in alignment may indicate mental retardation or a genitourinary malformation.

Remember to pull the pinna straight down on an infant or child under 3 years old. This method will match the slope of the ear canal.

When examining an infant or young child, a pneumatic bulb attachment enables you to direct a light puff of air toward the drum to assess vibratility (Fig. 8–5). For a secure seal, choose the largest speculum that will fit the ear canal without causing pain. A rubber tip on the end of the speculum gives a better seal. Give a small pump to the bulb (positive pressure), then release the bulb (negative pressure). Normally, the tympanic membrane moves inward with a slight puff and outward with a slight release.

An abnormal response is no movement of the eardrum. Drum hypomobility indicates effusion or a high vacuum in the middle ear. For the newborn's first 6 weeks, drum immobility is the best indicator of middle ear infection.

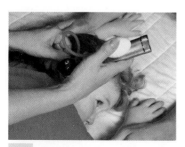

8–5   Using an otoscope with pneumatic bulb attachment.

Normal Range of Findings	Abnormal Findings
Normally, the tympanic membrane is intact. In a child being treated for chronic otitis media, you may note the presence of a tympanostomy tube in the central part of the drum. This is inserted surgically to equalize pressure and drain secretions. Note a foreign body in a child's ear canal, such as a small stone or bead.	Foreign body (see Table 15–3, p. 367, in Jarvis: *Physical Examination and Health Assessment,* 5th ed.).

The Aging Adult

Earlobes may be pendulous with linear wrinkling. Coarse, wiry hairs may be present at the opening of the ear canal. During otoscopy, the drum may normally be whiter in color and more opaque—duller than in the younger adult. It also may look thickened.

A high-tone frequency hearing loss is apparent for those affected with **presbycusis,** the hearing loss that occurs with aging. This condition is revealed by difficulty hearing whispered words in the voice test and difficulty hearing consonants during conversational speech.

For more information on assessment of the ears and hearing, see Chapter 15 in Jarvis: *Physical Examination and Health Assessment,* 5th ed., pp. 343-372.

Summary Checklist

For a PDA-downloadable version go to http://evolve.elsevier.com/Jarvis.

1. Inspect external ear:
Size and shape of auricle
Position and alignment on head
Skin condition
Color, lumps, lesions
Movement of auricle and tragus
(for tenderness)
External auditory meatus
Size, swelling, redness, discharge, cerumen, lesions, foreign bodies

2. Otoscopic examination:
External canal
Cerumen, discharge, foreign bodies, lesions

Redness or swelling of canal wall
Inspect tympanic membrane:
Color and characteristics
Note position (flat, bulging, retracted)
Integrity of membrane (no perforations)

3. Test hearing acuity:
Note behavioral response to conversational speech
Voice test
Tuning fork tests
Weber and Rinne tests

Nursing Diagnoses Commonly Associated With The Ears And Hearing Disorders

Impaired verbal **Communication**
Risk for **Infection**
Pain
Disturbed **Sensory** perception: auditory

Impaired **Social** interaction
Risk for **Trauma** related to balance difficulties

ABNORMAL FINDINGS

TABLE 8-1	Abnormalities of the Ear Canal or Tympanic Membrane

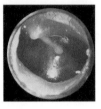

Retracted Drum

Landmarks look more prominent. Malleus handle looks shorter and more horizontal. Short process is very prominent. Light reflex is absent or distorted. Drum is dull and lusterless and does not move. Signs indicate obstructed eustachian tube and serous otitis media.

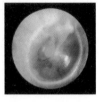

Otitis Media with Effusion

An amber-yellow drum, an air/fluid level with fine black dividing line, or air bubbles visible behind drum. Symptoms are feeling of fullness, transient hearing loss, popping sound with swallowing. Also called serous otitis media and glue ear.

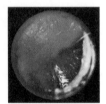

Acute (Purulent) Otitis Media

An absent or distorted light reflex is an early sign. Redness and bulging are first noted in superior part of drum (pars flaccida), along with earache and fever. Then fiery red bulging of entire drum occurs, with deep throbbing pain; fever; transient hearing loss. Pneumatic otoscopy reveals drum hypomobility.

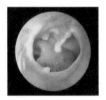

Perforation

Drum rupture from increased pressure or from trauma. Usually, perforation appears as a round or oval darkened area on the drum, but in this photo the perforation is very large. *Central* perforations occur in the pars tensa, *marginal* perforations at the annulus.

TABLE 8-1   Abnormalities of the Ear Canal or Tympanic Membrane

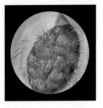

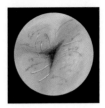

Excessive Cerumen

Excessive cerumen is produced or is impacted because of a narrow tortuous canal or faulty cleaning method. It may appear as a round ball partially obscuring the drum or totally occluding the canal. With total occlusion, the person experiences ear fullness and impaired hearing.

Otitis Externa

Severe swelling of canal; inflammation; tenderness. Here, canal lumen is narrowed to one-quarter its normal size. An infection of the outer ear, with severe painful movement of pinna and tragus, redness and swelling of pinna and canal, scanty purulent discharge, scaling, itching, fever, and enlarged tender regional lymph nodes. Hearing is normal or slightly diminished. More common in hot, humid weather; also called swimmer's ear. Canal becomes waterlogged and swells; skinfolds are set up for infection.

Chapter Nine

Nose, Mouth, and Throat

ANATOMY

The **nose** is the first segment of the respiratory system. It warms, moistens, and filters the inhaled air, and it is the sensory organ for smell.

The oval openings at the base of the nose are the *nares* (Fig. 9–1). The *columella* divides the two nares and is continuous inside with the nasal septum.

Inside, the **nasal cavity** is large and extends back over the roof of the mouth (Fig. 9–2). Nasal mucosa appears redder than oral mucosa because of the rich blood supply present to warm the inhaled air.

The lateral walls of each nasal cavity contain three bony projections—the *turbinates*. They increase the surface area so that more blood vessels are available to warm, humidify, and filter the inhaled air.

The **mouth** is the first segment of the digestive system and an airway for the respiratory system (Fig. 9–3). It contains the teeth and gums, tongue, and three pairs of salivary glands. The hard (bony) palate is whitish; the more posterior soft palate is an arch of muscle that is pinker and mobile.

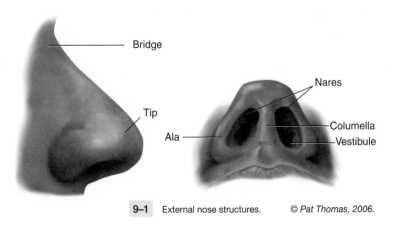

9–1   External nose structures.   © *Pat Thomas, 2006.*

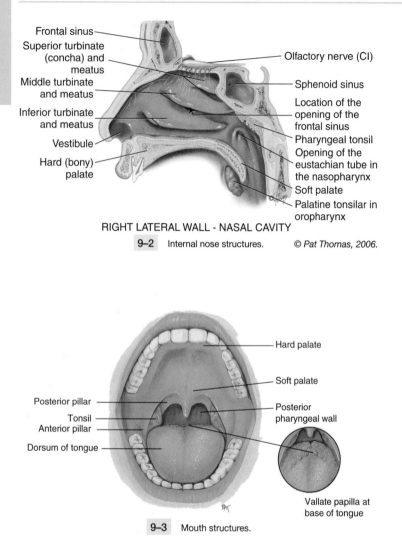

RIGHT LATERAL WALL - NASAL CAVITY

9-2   Internal nose structures.   © Pat Thomas, 2006.

9-3   Mouth structures.

🌐 **CROSS-CULTURAL CARE**

Bifid uvula, a condition in which the uvula is split either completely or partially, is common in Native American groups and Asians and is rare in whites and blacks.

Cleft lip and **cleft palate** are most common in Asians and Native Americans and least common in blacks. **Torus palatinus,** a bony ridge running in the middle of the hard palate, is common in Native Americans and in Inuits and Asians.

SUBJECTIVE DATA

Nose
1. Discharge
2. Frequent colds (upper respiratory infections)
3. Sinus pain
4. Trauma
5. Epistaxis (nosebleeds)
6. Allergies
7. Altered smell

Mouth and Throat
8. Sores or lesions
9. Sore throat
10. Bleeding gums
11. Toothache
12. Hoarseness
13. Dysphagia
14. Altered taste
15. Smoking, alcohol consumption
16. Self-care behaviors (dental care pattern, dentures or appliances)

OBJECTIVE DATA

PREPARATION

Position the person sitting up straight with his or her head at your eye level. Remove dentures.

EQUIPMENT NEEDED

Otoscope with short, wide-tipped nasal speculum attachment or nasal speculum and penlight
Tongue blade
Cotton gauze pad (4 × 4 inches)
Gloves

Normal Range of Findings	Abnormal Findings
Inspect and Palpate the Nose The nose is symmetric, in the midline, and in proportion to other facial features. Inspect for any deformity, asymmetry, inflammation, or skin lesions. Test the patency of the nostrils. This reveals any obstruction, which can later be explored using the nasal speculum.	 Absence of sniff indicates obstruction, e.g., nasal polyps, rhinitis.
Nasal Cavity Attach the short, wide-tipped speculum to the otoscope head and insert into the nasal vestibule, avoiding pressure on the nasal septum (Fig. 9–4). Inspect the nasal mucosa, noting its normal red color and smooth moist surface (Fig. 9–5). Note any swelling, discharge, bleeding, or foreign body.	 *Rhinitis*—Nasal mucosa is swollen and bright red with an upper respiratory infection.

Normal Range of Findings	Abnormal Findings

Discharge is common with rhinitis and sinusitis, varying from watery and copious to thick, purulent, and green-yellow.

With chronic allergy, mucosa looks swollen, boggy, pale, and gray.

For more information and illustrations on abnormalities of the nose, see Table 16–1, p. 398 in Jarvis: *Physical Examination and Health Assessment,* 5th ed.

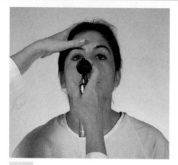

9–4   Viewing the naris through nasal speculum.

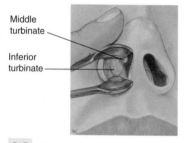

Middle turbinate

Inferior turbinate

9–5   Viewing the naris through nasal speculum.

Observe the nasal septum for deviation, perforation, or bleeding. A deviated septum is common and not significant unless airflow is obstructed.

A deviated septum looks like a hump or shelf in one nasal cavity.

Perforation is seen as a spot of light from penlight shining in other naris.

Epistaxis commonly comes from the anterior septum.

Inspect the turbinates, the bony ridges curving down from the lateral walls. The middle and inferior turbinates appear the same light red color as the nasal mucosa. Note any swelling but do not try to push the speculum past it. Turbinates are quite vascular and tender if touched.

Note any polyps, benign growths that accompany chronic allergy, and distinguish them from normal turbinates.

Polyps are smooth, pale gray, avascular, mobile, and nontender.

Normal Range of Findings	Abnormal Findings

Palpate the Sinus Areas

Using your thumbs, press over the frontal sinuses below the eyebrows and over the maxillary sinuses below the cheekbones. Do not press directly on the eyeballs. The person should feel firm pressure but no pain.

Sinus areas are tender to palpation in persons with chronic allergies and acute infection (sinusitis).

Inspect the Mouth

Lips

Inspect the lips for color, moisture, cracking, or lesions. Black persons may have bluish lips, which is normal.

In light-skinned people, circumoral pallor occurs with shock and anemia, cyanosis with hypoxemia and chilling, cherry red lips with carbon monoxide poisoning, acidosis from aspirin poisoning, or ketoacidosis.

Cheilitis (perleche)—cracking at the corners.

Herpes simplex, other lesions (Table 9–1 on p. 100).

Teeth and Gums

Teeth normally appear white, straight, evenly spaced, and clean and free of debris or decay. Note any diseased, absent, loose, or abnormally positioned teeth.

Discolored teeth—appear brown with excessive fluoride use, yellow with tobacco use.

Grinding down of tooth surface.

Plaque—Soft debris.
Caries—Decay.

Ask the person to bite, and note alignment of upper and lower jaw. Normal occlusion in the back is the upper teeth resting directly on the lowers; in the front, the upper incisors slightly override the lower incisors.

Malocclusion, e.g., protrusion of upper or lower incisors.

Normally, the gums look pink or coral with a stippled (dotted) surface. The gum margins are tight and well defined. Check for swelling, retraction of gingival margins, and spongy, bleeding, or discolored gums. Black people normally may have a dark, melanotic line along the gingival margin.

Gingival hypertrophy, crevices between teeth and gums, pockets of debris.

Gums bleed with slight pressure, indicating gingivitis.

Dark line on gingival margins occurs with lead and bismuth poisoning.

Tongue

The tongue color is pink and even. The dorsal surface is normally roughened from the papillae. A thin white coating may be present. Ask the person to touch the tongue to the roof of

Beefy red swollen tongue.
Smooth glossy areas (see Table 16–5, p. 403, in Jarvis: *Physical Examination and Health Assessment*, 5th ed.).

Normal Range of Findings	Abnormal Findings
the mouth. Its ventral surface looks smooth, glistening, and shows veins. Saliva is present.	Enlarged tongue occurs with mental retardation, hypothyroidism, acromegaly. Dry mouth occurs with dehydration, fever; tongue has deep vertical fissures. Excessive saliva and drooling.
Carefully inspect the tongue and the entire U-shaped area under the tongue. Note any white patches, nodules, or ulcerations. If lesions are present or with any person over 50 or with a positive history of smoking or alcohol use, put on a glove and palpate the area. Notice any induration.	Any lesion or ulcer persisting for more than 2 weeks must be investigated. An indurated area may be a mass or lymphadenopathy and must be investigated.
Buccal Mucosa The buccal mucosa looks pink, smooth, and moist, although patchy hyperpigmentation is common and normal in dark-skinned people.	Dappled brown patches are pres-ent with Addison's disease (chronic adrenal insufficiency).
Stensen's duct, the opening of the parotid salivary gland, looks like a small dimple opposite the upper second molar. You may also see a raised occlusion line on the buccal mucosa parallel with the level the teeth meet; this is due to the teeth closing against the cheek.	Orifice of Stensen's duct looks red with mumps. *Koplik's spots*—Small blue-white spots are a prodromal sign of measles.
Fordyce's granules are small, isolated white or yellow papules on the mucosa of the cheek, tongue, and lips. These little sebaceous cysts are painless and not significant.	The chalky white raised patch of *leukoplakia* is precancerous (see Table 16–4, p. 402, in Jarvis: *Physical Examination and Health Assessment,* 5th ed.).
Palate The more anterior hard palate is white with irregular transverse rugae. The posterior soft palate is pink, smooth, and upwardly movable. A common variation is a nodular bony ridge down the middle of the hard palate, a **torus palatinus** (see Table 9–1).	The hard palate appears yellow with jaundice. In blacks with jaundice, it may look yellow, muddy yellow, or green-brown. Oral *Kaposi's sarcoma* is a bruiselike, dark red, macular lesion, usually on the hard palate, that is a common early lesion with AIDS.
Ask the person to say "ahhh," and note the soft palate and uvula rise in the midline. This tests one function of cranial nerve X, the vagus nerve.	A *bifid* uvula appears as if split in two; it is more common in Native Americans (see Table 16–6, p. 405, in Jarvis: *Physical Examination and Health Assessment,* 5th ed.).

Normal Range of Findings	Abnormal Findings

Inspect the Throat

The **tonsils** are the same pink as the oral mucosa, and their surface is peppered with indentations or crypts. There should be no exudate on the tonsils. Tonsils are graded in size as:

1+: Visible
2+: Halfway between tonsillar pillars and uvula
3+: Touching the uvula
4+: Touching each other

You may normally see 1+ or 2+ tonsils in healthy people, especially in children.

Depress the tongue with a tongue blade. Scan the posterior pharyngeal wall for color, exudate, and lesions. When finished, discard the tongue blade.

Touching the posterior wall with the tongue blade elicits the gag reflex. This tests cranial nerves IX and X. Test cranial nerve XII, the hypoglossal nerve, by asking the person to stick out the tongue. It should protrude in the midline. Children enjoy this request. Note any tremor, loss of movement, or deviation to the side.

Notice any breath odor, *halitosis.* This is common and usually due to a local cause, such as poor oral hygiene, consumption of odoriferous foods, alcohol consumption, heavy smoking, or dental infection. Occasionally, it may indicate a systemic disease.

Abnormal Findings:

With an acute infection, tonsils are bright red, swollen, and may have exudate or large white spots. A white membrane covering the tonsils may accompany infectious mononucleosis, leukemia, and diphtheria.

Tonsils are enlarged to 2+, 3+, or 4+ with an acute infection.

With damage to cranial nerve XII, the tongue deviates toward the paralyzed side.

A fine tremor of the tongue occurs with hyperthyroidism, a coarse tremor with cerebral palsy and alcoholism.

Diabetic ketoacidosis has an accompanying sweet fruity breath odor; this acetone smell also occurs in children with malnutrition or dehydration. Others are an ammonia breath odor with uremia, a musty odor with liver disease, a foul, fetid odor with dental or respiratory infections, and alcohol odor with alcohol ingestion or chemicals.

♦ DEVELOPMENTAL CARE

Infants and Children

The newborn may have milia across the nose. The nasal bridge may be flat in black and Asian children. There should be no nasal flaring or narrowing with breathing.

Nasal flaring in the infant indicates respiratory distress.

In a child with chronic allergy, a transverse ridge is present across

Normal Range of Findings	Abnormal Findings
	the nose from wiping the nose up ward with the palm.
	Nasal narrowing on inhalation is seen with chronic nasal obstruction and mouth-breathing.
Note the number of teeth, and whether it is appropriate for the child's age. Also note patterns of eruption, position, condition, and hygiene. Use this guide for children under 2 years: The child's age in months minus the number 6 should equal the expected number of deciduous teeth. Normally, all 20 deciduous teeth are in by 2½ years.	No teeth by age 1 year. Discolored teeth—appear yellow or yellow-brown with infants taking tetracycline or whose mothers took the drug during the last trimester; appear green or black with excessive iron ingestion, although this reverses when the iron is stopped. Malocclusion—Upper or lower dental arches are out of alignment.
Note any bruising or laceration on the buccal mucosa or gums of infant or young child.	Trauma may indicate child abuse resulting from forced feeding of bottle or spoon.

The Pregnant Female

Gum hypertrophy (surface looks smooth and stippling disappears) may occur normally at puberty or during pregnancy (pregnancy gingivitis).

The Aging Adult

In the edentulous person, the mouth and lips fold in, giving a "pursestring" appearance. The teeth may look slightly yellowed, though the color is uniform. The teeth may look longer as the gum margins recede. Tooth surfaces look worn down or abraded.

The tongue looks smoother because of papillary atrophy. The aging adult's buccal mucosa is thinned and may look shinier as though it were varnished.

Old dental work deteriorates, especially at the gum margins. The teeth loosen with bone resorption and may move with palpation.

Summary Checklist

For a PDA-downloadable version go to http://evolve.elsevier.com/Jarvis.

Nose
1. **Inspect external nose:**
   Symmetry
   Deformity
   Lesions
2. **Palpate to test patency of each nostril**
3. **Inspect nasal cavity using nasal speculum:**
   Color and integrity of nasal mucosa
   Septum for deviation, perforation, or bleeding
   Turbinates, noting color, any exudate, swelling, or polyps
4. **Palpate the sinus areas for tenderness**

Mouth and Throat
1. **Inspect using penlight:**
   Lips, teeth and gums, tongue, buccal mucosa
   Color, intactness of structures, lesions
   Palate and uvula
   Integrity and mobility as person phonates
   Grade tonsils
   Pharyngeal wall
   Color, any exudate, or lesions
2. **Palpate mouth when indicated**

Nursing Diagnoses Commonly Associated with Nose, Mouth, Throat Disorders

Ineffective **Airway** clearance
Risk for **Aspiration**
Impaired verbal **Communication**
Impaired **Dentition**
Insomnia
Impaired **Oral** mucous membrane

Pain
Disturbed **Sensory** perception:
   olfactory
   gustatory
Impaired **Swallowing**

ABNORMAL FINDINGS

| TABLE 9-1 | Abnormalities of the Mouth and Throat |

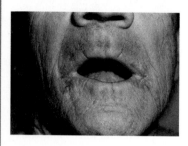

CHEILITIS (ANGULAR STOMATITIS, PERLECHE)

Erythema, scaling, shallow and painful fissures at the corners of the mouth occur with excess salivation and candidal infection. Seen in edentulous persons and those with poorly fitting dentures that cause folding in of corners of mouth.

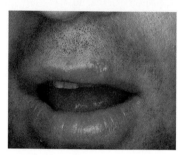

HERPES SIMPLEX I

Cold sores are groups of clear vesicles with a surrounding indurated erythematous base. These evolve into pustules, which rupture, weep, crust, and heal in 4 to 10 days. The most likely site is the lip–skin junction; infection often recurs in same site. Recurrent herpes simplex may be precipitated by sunlight, fever, colds, allergy.

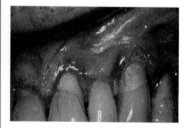

GINGIVITIS

Gum margins are red, swollen, and bleed easily. Note bulbous gingivae between the teeth. Inflammation is usually due to poor dental hygiene or vitamin C deficiency. The condition may occur in pregnancy and puberty as a result of a change in hormonal balance.

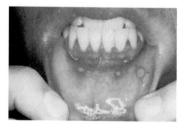

APHTHOUS ULCERS

A canker sore appears first as a vesicle, then as a small, round ulcer with a white base surrounded by a red halo. It is quite painful and lasts for 1 to 2 weeks. The cause is unknown, although it is associated with stress, fatigue, and food allergy.

TABLE 9-1 | Abnormalities of the Mouth and Throat

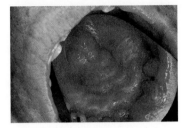

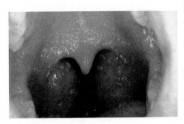

TORUS PALATINUS

A normal variation is a modular bony ridge down the middle of the hard palate (seen here using a mirror). This benign growth arises after puberty and is more common in Native Americans, Inuits, and Asians.

ACUTE TONSILLITIS AND PHARYNGITIS

Bright red throat, swollen tonsils, white or yellow exudate on tonsils and pharynx, swollen uvula, and enlarged, tender cervical and tonsillar nodes. Accompanied by severe sore throat, high fever of sudden onset. Caution: Cannot discriminate bacterial from viral infection on clinical data alone; all sore throats need a throat culture so as not to miss a *Streptococcus* infection.

Chapter 10

Breasts and Axillae, Including Regional Lymphatics

ANATOMY

The female **breasts** are accessory reproductive organs whose function is to produce milk. The breasts lie anterior to the pectoralis major and serratus anterior muscles, between the second and sixth ribs (Fig. 10–1). The superior lateral corner of breast tissue, called the **axillary tail of Spence,** projects up and laterally into the axilla.

The breast may be divided into four quadrants by imaginary horizontal and vertical lines intersecting at the nipple. This makes a convenient map to describe clinical findings: upper outer quadrant, lower outer, lower inner, and upper inner.

Internally, the breast is composed of (1) **glandular tissue,** containing 15 to 20 lobes radiating from the nipple (Fig. 10–2). Each lobe empties into a lactiferous duct and these converge toward the nipple. (2) The suspensory ligaments, or **Cooper's ligaments,** are fibrous bands extending vertically from the surface to the chest wall muscles. They support the breast. (3) The **adipose,** or fatty, tissue provides most of the bulk of the breast.

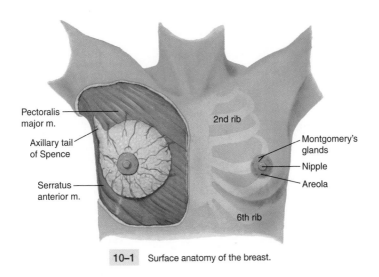

Pectoralis major m.

Axillary tail of Spence

Serratus anterior m.

2nd rib

Montgomery's glands

Nipple

Areola

6th rib

10–1 Surface anatomy of the breast.

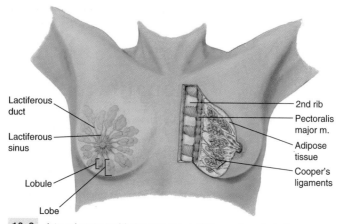

10–2   Internal anatomy: (1) glandular tissue, (2) fibrous tissue including suspensory ligaments, (3) adipose tissue.

The breast has extensive lymphatic drainage (Fig. 10–3): (1) **central axillary nodes,** high up in the middle of the axilla; (2) **pectoral** nodes, along the lateral edge of the pectoralis major muscle; (3) **subscapular** nodes, along the lateral edge of the scapula; (4) **lateral** nodes, along the humerus, inside the upper arm. From the central axillary nodes, drainage flows up to the infraclavicular and supraclavicular nodes.

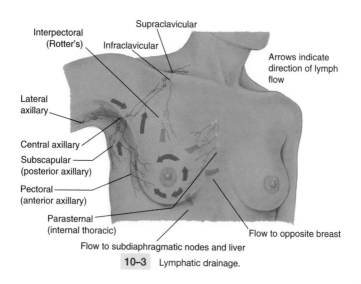

10–3   Lymphatic drainage.

CROSS-CULTURAL CARE

Racial differences in sexual maturity demonstrate that black girls begin puberty about 1 to 1.5 years earlier than white girls, and start menstruating about 8.5 months earlier (Herman-Giddens et al., 1997). The onset of breast development occurs at an average age of 8.87 years for black girls and 9.96 years for white girls (with Hispanic ethnicity occurring in both groups).

SUBJECTIVE DATA

BREAST
1. Pain
2. Lump
3. Discharge
4. Rash
5. Swelling
6. Trauma
7. History of breast disease
8. Surgery
9. Perform breast self-examination, last mammogram

AXILLA
10. Tenderness
11. Lump or swelling
12. Rash

OBJECTIVE DATA

PREPARATION
The woman is sitting up, facing you. Use a short gown, open at the back, and lift it up to the woman's shoulders during inspection. During palpation, the woman is supine; cover one breast with the gown while examining the other.

EQUIPMENT NEEDED
Small pillow
Ruler marked in centimeters
Pamphlet or teaching aid for breast self-examination

Normal Range of Findings	Abnormal Findings
Inspect the Breasts	
General Appearance	
Note symmetry of size and shape (common to have a slight asymmetry in size) (Fig. 10–4).	A sudden increase in size of one breast signifies trauma, inflammation, infection, or neoplasm.
Skin	
The skin is normally smooth and of even color with no redness, bulging, dimpling, skin lesions, or focal vascular pattern. A fine blue vascular network is normally visible in lightly pigmented females during pregnancy. Pale linear striae, or stretch marks, often follow pregnancy.	Hyperpigmentation. Redness and heat with inflammation. Unilateral dilated superficial veins in a nonpregnant woman.
Normally there is no edema.	Edema exaggerates the hair follicles, giving a "pig skin" or "orange peel" look (also called *peau d'orange*).

Normal Range of Findings	Abnormal Findings

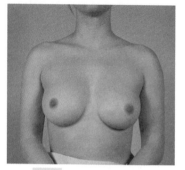

10–4   Breast appearance.

Lymphatic Drainage Areas

The axillary and supraclavicular regions have no bulging, discoloration, or edema.

Nipple

The nipples should be symmetrically located and usually protrude, although some are flat and some inverted. Distinguish a recently retracted nipple from one that has been inverted for many years or since puberty.

Note any dry scaling, any fissure or ulceration, and bleeding or other discharge. Normally, there are none.

A normal variation in about 1 percent of men and women is *supernumerary nipple*, a congenital finding. Usually, it is 5 to 6 cm below the breast near the midline and looks like a mole, although a close look reveals a tiny nipple and areola. It is not significant.

Maneuvers to Screen for Retraction

First ask the woman to lift arms slowly over her head. Both breasts should move up symmetrically.

Deviation in pointing.

Recent nipple retraction signifies acquired disease (see Table 17–3, p. 430, in Jarvis: *Physical Examination and Health Assessment,* 5th ed.).

Any discharge must be explored, especially in the presence of a breast mass.

Rarely, glandular tissue, a supernumerary breast, or polymastia, is present.

Retraction signs are due to fibrosis in the breast tissue, usually caused by growing neoplasms.

Note a lag in movement of one breast.

Normal Range of Findings	Abnormal Findings

Next ask her to put her hands onto her hips and push, and then to push her two palms together. There will be a slight lifting of both breasts.

Note a dimpling or a pucker that indicates skin retraction (see Table 17–3, p. 430, in Jarvis: *Physical Examination and Health Assessment*, 5th ed.).

Inspect and Palpate the Axillae

Inspect the skin, noting any rash or infection. Lift the woman's arm and support it yourself so that her muscles are loose and relaxed. Reach your fingers high into the axillae and move them firmly down in each direction.

Usually nodes are not palpable, although you may feel a small, soft, nontender node in the central group. Expect some tenderness when palpating high in the axillae. Note any enlarged and tender lymph nodes.

Nodes enlarge with any local infection of the breast, arm, or hand, and with breast cancer metastases.

Palpate the Breasts

Help the woman into a supine position. Tuck a small pad under the side to be palpated and raise her arm over her head to flatten the breast tissue and displace it medially.

Use the pads of your first three fingers and make a gentle rotary motion on the breast. Choose one of two patterns for palpation: (1) spokes-on-a-wheel (Fig. 10–5) (2) concentric circles (Fig. 10–6) or (3) vertical lines (Fig 10-7). Take care to palpate the tail of Spence extending from the upper quadrant into the axillae.

In nulliparous women, normal breast tissue feels firm, smooth, and elastic. After pregnancy, the tissue feels softer and looser. Premenstrual engorgement is normal due to increasing progesterone and consists of a slight enlargement, a tenderness to palpation, and a generalized nodularity; the lobes feel prominent and their margins are more distinct.

A firm transverse ridge of compressed tissue in the lower quadrants,

Heat, redness, and swelling in nonlactating and nonpostpartum breasts indicate inflammation.

Normal Range of Findings	Abnormal Findings

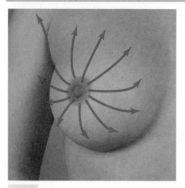

10–5 Spokes-on-a-wheel pattern of palpation.

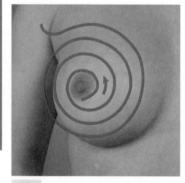

10–6 Concentric circles pattern of palpation.

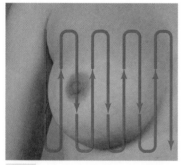

10–7 Vertical lines pattern of palpation.

Normal Range of Findings	Abnormal Findings
the **inframammary ridge,** is especially noticeable in large breasts. Do not confuse it with an abnormal lump.	
Palpate the nipple. Note any induration or subareolar masses. Use your thumb and forefinger to apply gentle pressure or a stripping action to the nipple. If any discharge appears, note its color and consistency. Pressing a white gauze pad to the discharge helps to determine its color.	Except in pregnancy and lactation, discharge is abnormal (see Table 17–6, p. XXX, in Jarvis: *Physical Examination and Health Assessment,* 5th ed.).
If you feel a lump or mass, note these characteristics:	See Table 10–1 on p. 113 for description of common breast lumps using these characteristics.

   1. Location—Diagram the breast in the woman's record and mark the location of the lump
   2. Size—In centimeters: width × length × thickness
   3. Shape—Oval, round, lobulated, or indistinct
   4. Consistency—Soft, firm, or hard
   5. Movable—Freely movable or fixed
   6. Distinctness—Solitary or multiple
   7. Nipple—Displaced or retracted
   8. Skin over the lump—Erythematous, dimpled, or retracted
   9. Tenderness—To palpation
   10. Lymphadenopathy

Teach Breast Self-Examination (BSE)

Help each woman establish a regular schedule of self-care. The best time to conduct BSE is right after the menstrual period, or the 4th through 7th day of the menstrual cycle, when the breasts are the smallest and least congested. Advise pregnant or menopausal women who are not having menstrual periods to select a familiar date to examine the breasts each month, such as their birth date.

Normal Range of Findings	Abnormal Findings

Describe the correct technique, rationale, and expected findings. Teach the woman to do this in front of a mirror while she is disrobed to the waist. At home, she can start palpation in the shower, where soap and water assist palpation. Palpation should then be performed while lying supine. Encourage the woman to palpate her own breasts while you are there to monitor her technique. Use the return demonstration to assess her technique and understanding of the procedure.

The Male Breast

Inspect the chest wall, noting the skin surface and any lumps or swelling. Palpate the nipple area for any lumps or tissue enlargement. It should feel even with no nodules.

The normal male breast has a flat disc of undeveloped breast tissue beneath the nipple. **Gynecomastia** is an enlargement of this breast tissue, making it clinically distinguishable from the other tissue in the chest wall. It feels like a smooth, firm, movable disc. This occurs normally during puberty. It usually affects only one breast and is temporary.

Gynecomastia also occurs with use of some medications and in some disease states (see Table 17–8, p. 435, in Jarvis: *Physical Examination and Health Assessment,* 5th ed.).

 ## DEVELOPMENTAL CARE

Infants and Children

In the neonate, the breasts may be enlarged and may secrete a clear or white fluid called "witch's milk." These signs are not significant and are resolved within a few days to a few weeks.

The Adolescent

Adolescent breast development usually begins between 9 and 13 years of age. Expect some asymmetry during

Note precocious development occurring before age 8. It is usually normal but also occurs with thyroid

Normal Range of Findings	Abnormal Findings

growth. Full development takes an average of 3 years, with a range of 1.5 to 6 years.

dysfunction, stilbestrol ingestion, or ovarian or adrenal tumor.

Note delayed development occurring with hormonal failure, anorexia nervosa beginning before puberty, or severe malnutrition.

With the maturing adolescent, palpate the breasts as you would with the adult. The breasts normally feel firm and uniform. Note any mass.

At this age, a mass is usually a benign fibroadenoma or a cyst.

The Pregnant Female

A delicate, blue vascular pattern is visible over the breasts of lightly pigmented females. The breasts increase in size as do the nipples. Jagged linear stretch marks, or *striae,* may develop if the breasts have a marked increase in size. The nipples also become darker and more erect. The areolae widen, grow darker, and contain small, scattered, elevated Montgomery's glands. On palpation, the breasts feel more nodular, and thick yellow colostrum can be expressed after the first trimester.

The Lactating Female

Colostrum changes to milk production around the third postpartum day. At this time, the breasts may become engorged; appear enlarged, reddened, and shiny; and feel warm and hard. Frequent nursing helps drain the ducts and sinuses and stimulates milk production.

Nipple soreness is normal, appears around the twentieth nursing day, lasts 24 to 48 hours, then disappears rapidly. The nipples may look red and irritated, and may even crack, but they heal rapidly if kept dry and exposed to air. Again, frequent nursing is the best treatment for nipple soreness.

One section of the breast surface appearing red and tender indicates a plugged duct (see Table 17–7, p. 434, in Jarvis: *Physical Examination and Health Assessment,* 5th ed.).

Normal Range of Findings	Abnormal Findings

The Aging Female

The breasts look pendulous, flattened, and sagging. Nipples may be retracted but can be pulled outward. The breasts feel more granular, and the terminal ducts around the nipple feel more prominent and stringy. Thickening of the inframammary ridge at the lower breast is normal and feels more prominent with age.

Reinforce the value of breast self-examination. Women over 50 years of age have an increased risk of breast cancer (Table 10–2, p. 115).

Because atrophy causes shrinkage of normal glandular tissue, cancer detection is somewhat easier. Any woman with a palpable lump not positively identified as a normal structure should be referred to a specialist.

Summary Checklist

For a PDA-downloadable version go to http://evolve.elsevier.com/Jarvis.

1. Inspection:
Inspect breasts as the woman sits, raises arms over head, pushes hands on hips, leans forward
Inspect the supraclavicular and infraclavicular areas

2. Palpation:
Palpate the axillae and regional lymph nodes
With woman supine, palpate the breast tissue, including the tail of Spence, the nipples, and the areolae

3. Teaching:
Teach breast self-examination

Nursing Diagnoses Commonly Associated with Breast Disorders

Anxiety
Disturbed **Body** image
Ineffective **Breastfeeding**
Interrupted **Breastfeeding**
Ineffective **Coping**

Grieving
Deficient **Knowledge:** breast self-examination
Risk for **Loneliness**
Pain

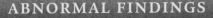

ABNORMAL FINDINGS

TABLE 10–1	Breast Lump

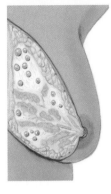

BENIGN BREAST DISEASE

(Formerly fibrocystic breast disease) Multiple tender masses. *Fibrocystic breast disease* is no longer a useful term because it covers too many entities. There are actually six diagnostic categories, based on symptoms and physical findings:

- Swelling and tenderness (cyclic discomfort)
- Mastalgia (severe pain, both cyclic and noncyclic)
- Nodularity (significant lumpiness, both cyclic and noncyclic)
- Dominant lumps (including cysts and fibroadenomas)
- Nipple discharge (including intraductal papilloma and duct ectasia)
- Infections and inflammations (including subareolar abscess, lactational mastitis, breast abscess, and Mondor's disease) (Love, 2000)

About 50% of all women have some form of benign breast disease. Nodularity occurs bilaterally; nodules are regular, firm, mobile, well demarcated, and rubbery, like small water balloons. Pain may be dull, heavy, and cyclic or may occur just before menses as nodules enlarge. Some women have nodularity but no pain or vice versa. Cysts are discrete, fluid-filled sacs. Dominant lumps and nipple discharge must be investigated carefully and may need to undergo biopsy to rule out cancer. Nodularity itself is not premalignant but may produce difficulty in detecting other cancerous lumps.

Continued

TABLE 10–1	Breast Lump—cont'd

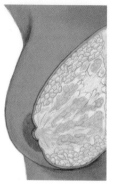 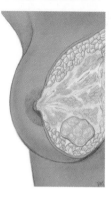

CANCER

Solitary unilateral nontender mass. Single focus in one area, although it may be interspersed with other nodules. Solid, hard, dense, and fixed to underlying tissues or skin as cancer becomes invasive. Borders are irregular and poorly delineated. Grows constantly. Often painless, although the person may have pain. Most common in upper outer quadrant. Usually found in women aged 30 to 80; increased risk in ages 40 to 44 and in women older than 50 years. As cancer advances, signs include firm or hard irregular axillary nodes, skin dimpling, nipple retraction, elevation, and discharge.

FIBROADENOMA

Solitary nontender mass. A category of benign breast disease that deserves mention because of its frequency and characteristic appearance. Solid, firm, rubbery, and elastic. Round, oval, or lobulated; 1 to 5 cm. Freely movable, slippery; fingers slide it easily through tissue. Most common in younger women between 15 and 30 years but can occur up to age 55 years. Grows quickly and constantly. Benign, although it must be diagnosed by biopsy.

TABLE 10–2　Breast Cancer Risk Factors

Risk Factors that Cannot be Changed	Lifestyle-Related Risk Factors
Female gender, age >50	Nulliparity or first child after age 30
Personal history of breast cancer	Recent oral contraceptive use
Mutation of BRCA1 and BRCA2 genes	Postmenopausal hormone therapy/ especially
First-degree relative with breast cancer (mother, sister, daughter)	Not breast-feeding
Previous breast biopsy with *atypical hyperplasia*, or *breast disease without atypia* or *usual hyperplasia*	Alcohol intake of ≥ 1 drink daily
Previous breast irradiation	Obesity (especially after menopause) and high-fat diet
Menstruation before age 12 or menopause after age 50	Physical inactivity

Data adapted from American Cancer Society: http://www.cancer.org/docroot/CRI/content/CRI_2_4_2X_What_are_the_risk_factors_for_breast_cancer_5.asp

Thorax and Lungs

ANATOMY

The **thoracic cage** is a bony structure with a conical shape (Fig. 11–1). It is defined by the sternum, 12 pairs of ribs, 12 thoracic vertebrae, and the diaphragm.

The *costochondral junctions* are the points at which the ribs join their cartilages. They are not palpable.

The *suprasternal notch* is the hollow U-shaped depression just above the sternum, between the clavicles.

The *manubriosternal angle,* or angle of Louis, is the articulation of the manubrium and body of the sternum, and it is continuous with the second rib. Each intercostal space is numbered by the rib above it.

The *costal angle* is formed by the right and left costal margins where

they meet at the xiphoid process. It is usually 90 degrees or less.

The **trachea** lies anterior to the esophagus and is 10 to 11 cm long in adults (Fig. 11–2). It begins at the level of the cricoid cartilage in the neck and bifurcates just below the sternal angle into the right and left main bronchi.

An **acinus** is a functional respiratory unit and consists of the bronchioles and alveoli. Gaseous exchange occurs across the respiratory membrane in the alveolar duct and in the millions of alveoli.

In the **anterior chest,** the *apex,* or highest point, of lung tissue is 3 or 4 cm above the inner third of the clavicles (Fig. 11–3). The *base,* or lower border,

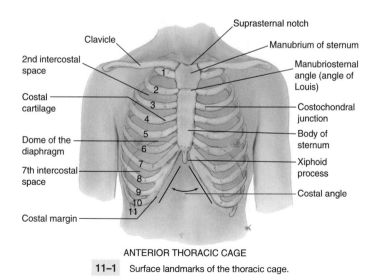

ANTERIOR THORACIC CAGE

11–1 Surface landmarks of the thoracic cage.

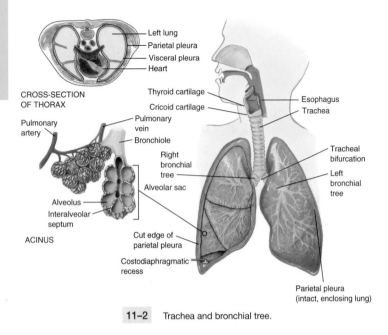

CROSS-SECTION OF THORAX

— Left lung
— Parietal pleura
— Visceral pleura
— Heart

Thyroid cartilage
Cricoid cartilage

Esophagus
Trachea

Pulmonary artery
Pulmonary vein
Bronchiole

Right bronchial tree
Alveolar sac

Tracheal bifurcation
Left bronchial tree

Alveolus
Interalveolar septum

ACINUS

Cut edge of parietal pleura
Costodiaphragmatic recess

Parietal pleura (intact, enclosing lung)

11–2   Trachea and bronchial tree.

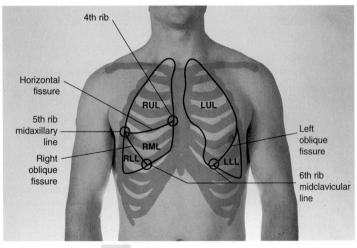

4th rib

Horizontal fissure

5th rib midaxillary line

Right oblique fissure

RUL   LUL

RML

RLL   LLL

Left oblique fissure

6th rib midclavicular line

11–3   Lobes of the lungs—anterior.

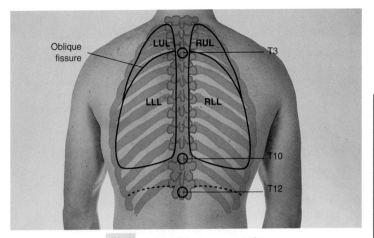

11–4   Lobes of the lungs—posterior.

rests on the diaphragm. The right lung has three lobes, and the left lung has two lobes. The lobes are separated by fissures.

Posteriorly, the location of the seventh cervical vertebra (C7) marks the apex of lung tissue and T10 usually corresponds to the base (Fig. 11–4). The most remarkable point about the posterior chest is that it is almost all lower lobe. The upper lobes occupy only a small band of tissue from the apices down to T3 or T4. The rest is all lower lobe. The right middle lobe does not project onto the posterior chest.

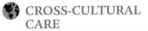 **CROSS-CULTURAL CARE**

Biocultural differences occur in the size of the thoracic cavity. In descending order, the largest chest volumes are found in whites, blacks, Asians, and Native Americans. Even considering the shorter height of Asians, their chest volume remains significantly lower than in whites and blacks.

The incidence of **tuberculosis** (TB) is higher in those who have recently immigrated to the United States from countries with a high endemic rate of TB including Mexico, the Philippines, Vietnam, India, and China (CDC, 2004).

SUBJECTIVE DATA

1. Cough (duration, productive of sputum)
2. Shortness of breath (with level of activity)
3. Chest pain with breathing
4. Past history of respiratory disease (bronchitis, emphysema, asthma, pneumonia, tuberculosis)
5. Smoking history (number of packs per day, number of years smoked)
6. Environmental exposure that affects breathing (e.g., occupational hazard or urban environment)
7. Self-care behaviors (last tuberculin skin test, chest x-ray, influenza immunization)

OBJECTIVE DATA

PREPARATION

Ask the person to sit upright and males to disrobe to the waist. Leave the gown on females open at the back.

EQUIPMENT NEEDED

Stethoscope
Small ruler marked in centimeters
Marking pen
Alcohol wipe (to clean endpiece)

Normal Range of Findings	Abnormal Findings

Inspect the Posterior Chest

Shape and Configuration. The spinous processes are in a straight line. The thorax is symmetric with downward sloping ribs. The scapulae are placed symmetrically.

The anteroposterior diameter of the chest is less than the transverse diameter. The ratio of anteroposterior to transverse diameter is 1:2 to 5:7.

The neck muscles and trapezius muscles are developed normally for age and occupation.

Position. This includes a relaxed posture with arms comfortably at the sides or hands in the lap.

Skin Color and Condition. Color should be consistent with person's genetic background, with no cyanosis or pallor. Note any lesions.

Palpate the Posterior Chest

Symmetric Expansion. Confirm *symmetric chest expansion* by placing your warmed hands on the posterolateral chest wall with thumbs at the level of T9 or T10. Slide your hands medially to pinch up a small fold of skin between your thumbs. Ask the person to take a deep breath; your thumbs should move apart symmetrically. Note any lag in expansion.

When severe, skeletal deformities may limit thoracic cage excursions, including scoliosis (S-shaped curvature) and kyphosis (outward curvature) of the thoracic spine.

Anteroposterior diameter that is equal to transverse diameter, or "barrel chest," with ribs horizontal, occurs in chronic emphysema due to hyperinflation of the lungs.

Neck muscles are hypertrophied in chronic obstructive pulmonary disease (COPD) from aiding in forced respirations.

With COPD, a tripod position (leaning forward with arms braced against knees, chair, or bed) gives leverage so that the rectus abdominis, intercostal, and accessory neck muscles can aid in expiration.

Unequal chest expansion occurs with marked atelectasis or pneumonia, with thoracic trauma such as fractured ribs, or with pneumothorax.

Pain accompanies deep breathing when the pleurae are inflamed.

Normal Range of Findings	Abnormal Findings

Tactile Fremitus. *Tactile fremitus* is a palpable vibration. Use the palmar base (the ball) of the fingers of one hand and touch the person's chest while he or she repeats the words "ninety-nine" or "blue moon." Start over the lung apices and palpate from one side to another; the vibrations should feel the same in the corresponding area on each side.

Normally, fremitus is most prominent between the scapulae and around the sternum, sites where the major bronchi are closest to the chest wall. Fremitus normally decreases as you progress down because more and more tissue impedes sound transmission.

Chest Wall. Using the fingers, gently *palpate the entire chest wall.* Note any areas of tenderness, increased skin temperature and moisture, any superficial lumps or masses, and any skin lesions.

Decreased fremitus occurs when anything obstructs transmission of vibrations, e.g., obstructed bronchus, pleural effusions or thickening, pneumothorax, or emphysema.

Increased fremitus occurs with compression or consolidation of lung tissue, e.g., lobar pneumonia (see Table 18–5, p. 470, in Jarvis: *Physical Examination and Health Assessment,* 5th ed.).

Crepitus is a coarse, crackling sensation palpable over the skin surface. It occurs in subcutaneous emphysema when air escapes from the lung and enters the subcutaneous tissue, as after open thoracic injury or surgery.

Percuss the Posterior Chest

Lung Fields. Start at the apices and percuss in the interspaces: make a side-to-side comparison all the way down the lung region. Percuss at 5-cm intervals. Avoid the scapulae and ribs.

Resonance predominates in healthy lung tissue in the adult. The resonant note may be modified somewhat in athletes with heavily muscular chest walls and in heavily obese adults in whom subcutaneous fat produces scattered dullness.

Diaphragmatic Excursion. Percuss to map out the lower lung border, both in expiration and inspiration. Measure the difference. This *diaphragmatic excursion* should be equal bilaterally and measure about 3 to 5 cm in adults, although it may be up to 7 to 8 cm in well-conditioned people.

Hyperresonance is found when too much air is present, as in emphysema or pneumothorax.

A **dull** note signals abnormal density in the lungs, as with pneumonia, pleural effusion, atelectasis, or tumor.

An abnormally high level of dullness on the chest wall, as well as absence of excursion, occurs with pleural effusion or atelectasis of the lower lobes.

Normal Range of Findings	Abnormal Findings

Auscultate the Posterior Chest

Breath Sounds. Instruct the person to breathe through the mouth a little bit deeper than usual. While standing behind the person, listen to the following lung areas—posterior from the apices at C7 to the bases (around T10) and laterally from the axillae down to the seventh or eighth rib. Use the side-to-side sequence illustrated in Figure 11–5. You should expect to hear three types of normal breath sounds: **bronchial** (sometimes called tracheal or tubular), **bronchovesicular,** and **vesicular** (see Table 11–1 below).

TABLE 11–1	Characteristics of Normal Breath Sounds		
	Pitch	Amplitude	Duration
Bronchial (Tracheal)	High	Loud	Inspiration < expiration
Bronchovesicular	Moderate	Moderate	Inspiration = expiration
Vesicular	Low	Soft	Inspiration > expiration

Normal Range of Findings	Abnormal Findings

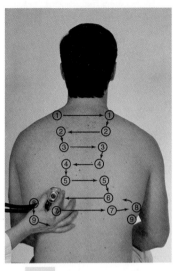

11–5   Order of auscultation.

Quality	Normal Location
Harsh, hollow, tubular	Trachea and larynx
Mixed	Over major bronchi where fewer alveoli are located: posterior, between scapulae, especially on right; anterior, around upper sternum in first and second intercostal spaces
Rustling like the sound of the wind in the trees	Over peripheral lung fields where air flows through smaller bronchioles and alveoli

Normal Range of Findings	Abnormal Findings

Note the normal location of the three types of breath sounds (Fig. 11–6; see also Fig. 11–7 on p. 126).

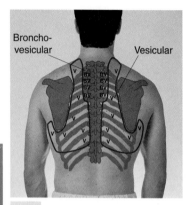

Broncho-vesicular

Vesicular

11–6   Breath sounds on the posterior chest.

Adventitious Sounds. Note the presence of any **adventitious sounds.** These are abnormal sounds caused by the collision of moving air with secretions in the tracheobronchial passageways or by the popping open of a previously deflated airway.

Inspect the Anterior Chest

Shape and Configuration. The ribs are sloping downward with symmetric interspaces. The costal angle is within 90 degrees. Development of abdominal muscles is as expected for the person's age, weight, and athletic condition.

Facial Expression. Relaxed and benign, indicating an unconscious effort of breathing.

Level of Consciousness. Alert and cooperative.

Decreased or absent breath sounds occur:

1. When the bronchial tree is obstructed by secretions, mucous plug, or a foreign body.
2. In emphysema due to loss of elasticity in the lung fibers and decreased force of inspired air.
3. When anything obstructs transmission of sound, such as pleurisy or pleural thickening, or air (pneumothorax) or fluid (pleural effusion) in the pleural space.

Increased breath sounds— Bronchial sounds are abnormal over the peripheral lung fields. They occur when consolidation (e.g., in pneumonia) or compression yields a denser lung area that enhances the transmission of sound from the bronchi. When the inspired air reaches the alveoli, it hits solid lung tissue, which conducts sound more efficiently to the surface.

Crackles (or rales) occur with pneumonia and pulmonary edema, and **wheezes** (or rhonchi) occur with asthma and emphysema (see Table 11–2 on p. 129).

Barrel chest has horizontal ribs and costal angle greater than 90 degrees.

Hypertrophy of abdominal muscles occurs with chronic emphysema.

Tense, strained, tired facies accompanies COPD.

Cerebral hypoxia may be reflected by excessive drowsiness or by anxiety, restlessness, and irritability.

Normal Range of Findings	Abnormal Findings

Skin Color and Condition. The lips and nail beds are free of cyanosis or unusual pallor. The nails are of normal configuration.

Quality of Respirations. Normal, relaxed breathing is automatic and effortless, regular, and even, and produces no noise. The chest expands symmetrically with each inspiration. Note any localized lag on inspiration.

Clubbing of distal fingertips occurs with chronic respiratory disease.

Noisy breathing occurs with severe asthma or chronic bronchitis.

Unequal chest expansion occurs when part of the lung is obstructed or collapsed, as with pneumonia, or with guarding to avoid postoperative incisional pain or the pain of pleurisy.

The rectus abdominis and internal intercostal muscles are used to force expiration in COPD.

The respiratory rate is within normal limits for the person's age, and the pattern of breathing is regular. Occasional sighs normally punctuate breathing.

Tachypnea and hyperventilation, bradypnea and hypoventilation, periodic breathing (see full description in Table 11–3 on p. 131).

Percuss the Anterior Chest

Begin at the apices. Percussing the interspaces and comparing one side to the other, move down the anterior chest.

Normally you hear a resonant note over healthy lung tissue. Note the borders of cardiac dullness normally found on the anterior chest, and do not confuse these with suspected lung pathology. In the right hemithorax, the upper border of liver dullness is located in the fifth intercostal space in the right midclavicular line. On the left, tympany is evident over the gastric space (see Fig. 18–24, p. 460, in Jarvis: *Physical Examination and Health Assessment,* 5th ed.).

Lungs are hyperinflated with chronic emphysema, resulting in hyperresonance where cardiac dullness would be expected.

Auscultate the Anterior Chest

Auscultate the lung fields over the anterior chest from the apices in the supraclavicular areas down to the sixth rib. Progress from side to side as you move downward, and listen to one full

Normal Range of Findings

respiration in each location. You should expect to hear vesicular breath sounds over most of the anterior lung fields as indicated in Figure 11–7.

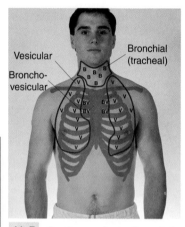

11–7   Breath sounds on the anterior chest.

🜲 DEVELOPMENTAL CARE

Infants and Children

Count the respiratory rate for 1 full minute, if possible, when the infant is asleep, because infants reach rapid rates with very little excitation when awake. The respiratory pattern may be irregular when there are extremes in room temperature or with feeding or sleeping. Brief periods of apnea less than 10 or 15 seconds are common. This periodic breathing is more common in premature infants.

Auscultation normally yields bronchovesicular breath sounds in the peripheral lung fields in the infant and young child up to age 5 or 6, because of the relatively thin chest wall with underdeveloped musculature.

Abnormal Findings

Rapid respiratory rates accompany pneumonia, fever, pain, heart disease, and anemia.

In an infant, tachypnea of 50 to 100 breaths per minute during sleep may be an early sign of congestive heart failure.

Diminished breath sounds occur with pneumonia, atelectasis, pleural effusion, or pneumothorax.

Normal Range of Findings	Abnormal Findings
Fine crackles are the adventitious sounds commonly heard in the immediate newborn period and are due to opening of the airways and clearing of fluid. Because the newborn's chest wall is so thin, transmission of sounds is enhanced and heard easily all over the chest, making localizations of breath sounds a problem. Even bowel sounds are easily heard in the chest. Try using the smaller pediatric diaphragm endpiece or place the bell over the infant's interspaces, not over the ribs.	Persistent fine crackles scattered over the chest occur with pneumonia, bronchiolitis, or atelectasis. Crackles only in upper lung fields occur with cystic fibrosis; crackles only in lower lung fields occur with heart failure. Expiratory wheezing occurs with asthma or bronchiolitis. Persistent peristaltic sounds with diminished breath sounds on the same side may indicate diaphragmatic hernia. Stridor is a high-pitched inspiratory crowing sound heard without the stethoscope that occurs with croup, acute epiglottitis, or foreign body aspiration.

The Pregnant Female

The thoracic cage may appear wider and the costal angle may feel wider than in the nonpregnant state. Respirations may be deeper.

The Aging Adult

The chest cage commonly shows an increased anteroposterior diameter, giving a round barrel shape and **kyphosis,** or an outward curvature of the thoracic spine. The person compensates by holding the head extended and tilted back.

You may palpate marked bony prominences because of decreased subcutaneous fat. Chest expansion may be somewhat decreased although still symmetric. The costal cartilages become calcified with age, resulting in a less mobile thorax.

An older person may fatigue easily, especially during auscultation when deep mouth-breathing is required. Take care that this person does not hyperventilate and become dizzy. Allow brief rest periods or quiet breathing. If the person does feel faint, holding the breath for a few seconds will restore equilibrium.

Summary Checklist

For a PDA-downloadable version go to http://evolve.elsevier.com/Jarvis.

1. **Inspection:**
   Thoracic cage
   Respirations
   Skin color and condition
   Person's position
   Facial expression
   Level of consciousness
2. **Palpation:**
   Confirm symmetric expansion
   Tactile fremitus
   Detect any lumps, masses,
      tenderness
3. **Percussion:**
   Percuss over lung fields
   Estimate diaphragmatic excursion
4. **Auscultation:**
   Assess normal breath sounds
   Note any abnormal breath sounds
   Note any adventitious sounds

Nursing Diagnoses Commonly Associated with the Thorax and Lungs—Respiratory Disorders

Activity intolerance
Ineffective **Airway** clearance
Anxiety
Ineffective **Breathing** pattern
Fatigue
Excess **Fluid** volume
Impaired **Gas** exchange
Impaired **Home** maintenance
Risk for **Infection**
Insomnia

Pain
Ineffective **Role** performance
Self-care deficit
Ineffective **Tissue** perfusion (renal,
   cardiopulmonary, cerebral,
   peripheral)
Impaired spontaneous **Ventilation**
Dysfunctional **Ventilatory** weaning
   response (DVWR)

ABNORMAL FINDINGS

TABLE 11–2 Adventitious Sounds*

Sound	Description	Mechanism	Clinical Example
(1) Discontinuous Sounds			
Crackles—fine (rales) Inspiration Expiration	Discontinuous, high-pitched, short, crackling, popping sounds heard during inspiration and that are not cleared by coughing.	Inhaled air collides with previously deflated airways: airways suddenly pop open, creating crackling sound.	*Late inspiratory crackles* occur with restrictive disease: pneumonia, congestive heart failure, and interstitial fibrosis. *Early inspiratory crackles* occur with obstructive disease: chronic bronchitis, asthma, and emphysema.
Crackles—coarse (coarse rales)	Loud, low-pitched, bubbling, and gurgling sounds that start in early inspiration and may be present in expiration	Inhaled air collides with secretions in the trachea and large bronchi.	Pulmonary edema, pneumonia, pulmonary fibrosis, and in the terminally ill who have a depressed cough reflex.
Atelectatic crackles (atelectatic rales)	Sound like fine crackles but do not last and are not pathologic. Disappear after the first few breaths. Heard in axillae and bases (usually dependent) of lungs.	When sections of alveoli are not fully aerated, they deflate and accumulate secretions. Crackles are heard when these sections reexpand with a few deep breaths.	In aging adults, bedridden persons, or in persons just roused from sleep.

*Although nothing in clinical practice seems to differ more than the nomenclature of adventitious sounds, most authorities concur on two categories: (1) discontinuous, discrete crackling sounds and (2) continuous, musical sounds

Continued

TABLE 11–2	Adventitious Sounds—cont'd		
Sound	Description	Mechanism	Clinical Example
Pleural friction rub	A very superficial sound that is coarse and low pitched; it has a grating quality as if two pieces of leather are being rubbed together. Sounds just like crackles, but *close* to the ear.	Caused when pleurae become inflamed and lose their normal lubricating fluid. Their opposing, roughened pleural surfaces rub together during respiration.	Pleuritis accompanied by pain with breathing. (Rub disappears after a few days if pleural fluid accumulates and separates pleurae.)

(2) Continuous Sounds

Wheeze—high pitched (sibilant)	High-pitched, musical, squeaking sounds that predominate in expiration but may occur in both expiration and inspiration.	Air squeezed or compressed through passageways narrowed almost to closure by collapsing, swelling, secretions, or tumors.	Obstructive lung disease such as asthma or emphysema
Wheeze—low pitched (sonorous rhonchi)	Low-pitched, musical snoring, moaning sounds. They are heard throughout the cycle, although they are more prominent on expiration. May clear somewhat by coughing.	Airflow obstruction. The pitch of the wheeze cannot be correlated to the size of the passageway that generates it.	Bronchitis
Stridor	High-pitched, monophonic, inspiratory crowing sound, louder in neck than over chest wall.	Originating in larynx or upper airway obstruction from swollen, inflamed tissues or lodged foreign body.	Croup, and acute epiglottitis in children, and foreign body inhalation. Obstructed airway may be life threatening.

TABLE 11–3 | Respiratory Patterns*

Inspiration   Expiration

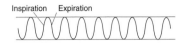

Normal Adult (for Comparison)

Rate—10 to 20 breaths per minute
Depth—500 to 800 ml
Pattern—even
The ratio of pulse to respiration is fairly
  constant, about 4:1. Both values increase
  as a normal response to exercise, fear, or
  fever.

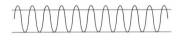

Sigh

Occasional sighs punctuate the normal
  breathing pattern and expand alveoli.
  Frequent sighs may indicate emotional dysfunction and may lead to
  hyperventilation and dizziness.

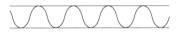

Tachypnea

Rapid shallow breathing. Increased
  rate >24 per minute. This is a normal
  response to fever, fear, or exercise. Rate
  also increases with respiratory insufficiency, pneumonia, alkalosis, pleurisy,
  and lesions in the pons.

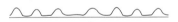

Hyperventilation

Increase in both rate and depth. Normally occurs with extreme exertion,
  fear, or anxiety. Also occurs with diabetic ketoacidosis (Kussmaul's respirations), hepatic coma, salicylate
  overdose, lesions of the midbrain,
  and alteration in blood gas
  concentration.

Bradypnea

Slow breathing. A decreased but regular
  rate (less than 10 per minute), as in
  drug-induced depression of the respiratory center in the medulla, increased intracranial pressure, and diabetic coma.

Hypoventilation

An irregular, shallow pattern caused by
  an overdose of narcotics or anesthet-
  ics and with prolonged bedrest or
  conscious splinting of the chest to
  avoid respiratory pain.

*Assess the (1) rate, (2) depth (tidal volume), and (3) pattern.   *Continued*

TABLE 11-3 | Respiratory Patterns—cont'd

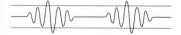 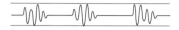

Cheyne-Stokes Respiration

A cycle in which respirations gradually increase in rate and depth and then decrease. The breathing periods last 30 to 45 seconds with periods of apnea (20 seconds) alternating the cycle. The most common cause is severe congestive heart failure; other causes are renal failure, meningitis, drug overdose, increased intracranial pressure. Occurs normally in infants and aging persons during sleep.

Biot's Respiration

Similar to Cheyne-Stokes respiration except that pattern is irregular. A series of normal respirations (three or four) is followed by a period of apnea. The cycle length is variable, lasting anywhere from 10 seconds to 1 minute. Seen with head trauma, brain abscess, heatstroke, spinal meningitis, and encephalitis.

Chapter Twelve

Heart and Neck Vessels

ANATOMY

The **precordium** is the area on the anterior chest overlying the heart and great vessels. The heart extends from the second to the fifth intercostal space, and from the right border of the sternum to the left midclavicular line (Fig. 12–1).

Think of the heart as an upside-down triangle in the chest. The "top" of the heart is the broader **base,** and the bottom is the **apex,** which points down and to the left. During contraction, the apex beats against the chest wall, producing an **apical impulse.**

The right side of the heart pumps blood into the lungs, and the left side of the heart simultaneously pumps blood into the body. Each side has an **atrium** and a **ventricle** (Fig. 12–2). The atrium is a thin-walled reservoir for holding blood, and the thick-walled ventricle is the muscular pumping chamber.

There are four **valves** in the heart. The two **atrioventricular** (AV) valves separate the atria and the ventricles. The right AV valve is the **tricuspid;** the left AV valve is the **bicuspid,** or

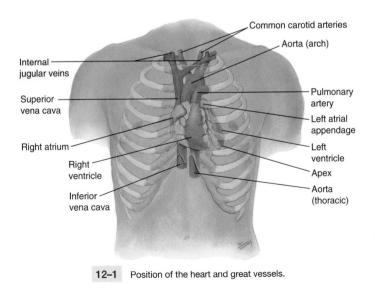

Internal jugular veins

Superior vena cava

Right atrium

Right ventricle

Inferior vena cava

Common carotid arteries

Aorta (arch)

Pulmonary artery

Left atrial appendage

Left ventricle

Apex

Aorta (thoracic)

12–1 Position of the heart and great vessels.

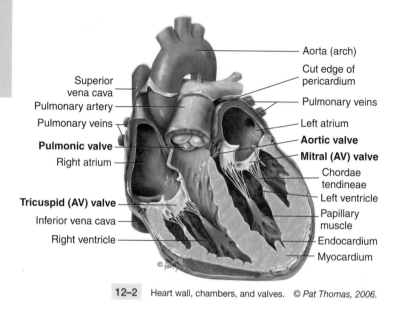

Aorta (arch)

Cut edge of pericardium

Pulmonary veins

Left atrium

Aortic valve

Mitral (AV) valve

Chordae tendineae

Left ventricle

Papillary muscle

Endocardium

Myocardium

Superior vena cava

Pulmonary artery

Pulmonary veins

Pulmonic valve

Right atrium

Tricuspid (AV) valve

Inferior vena cava

Right ventricle

12–2   Heart wall, chambers, and valves.   © Pat Thomas, 2006.

mitral, valve. The AV valves open during the heart's filling phase, or **diastole,** to allow the ventricles to fill with blood.

The **semilunar** (SL) valves are set between the ventricles and the arteries. The semilunar valves are the **pulmonic** valve in the right side of the heart and the **aortic** valve in the left side of the heart. They open during pumping, or **systole,** to allow blood to be ejected from the heart.

The **cardiac cycle** is the rhythmic movement of blood through the heart. It has two phases, **diastole** and **systole** (Fig. 12–3).

In **diastole,** the ventricles relax and fill with blood. The AV valves, the tricuspid and mitral, are open. During the first rapid filling phase, **protodiastolic filling,** blood pours rapidly from

the atria into the ventricles. Toward the end of diastole, the atria contract and push the last amount of blood into the ventricles, called **presystole.**

The closure of the AV valves contributes to the first heart sound (S_1) and signals the beginning of **systole.** The AV valves close to prevent any regurgitation of blood back up into the atria during contraction. Then the semilunar valves, the aortic and pulmonic, open, and blood is ejected rapidly into the arteries.

After the ventricles' contents are ejected, the semilunar valves close. This causes the second heart sound (S_2) and signals the end of systole.

Cardiovascular assessment includes the neck vessels—the carotid artery and the jugular veins (Fig. 12–4).

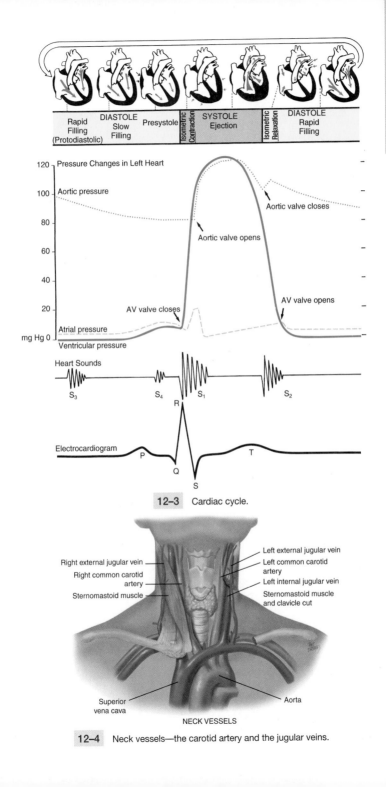

12–3 Cardiac cycle.

NECK VESSELS

12–4 Neck vessels—the carotid artery and the jugular veins.

CROSS-CULTURAL CARE

Heart disease and stroke account for more than one-third of all deaths among individuals from culturally diverse backgrounds. Under age 35, heart disease mortality for Native Americans is approximately twice as high as that for all other Americans. Black men are nearly twice as likely to die of stroke as white men, and their death rate related to stroke is more than double that of other ethnic groups.

Blacks have a higher incidence of hypertension than whites. The prevalence in blacks is 43% for adult males, 47% for females, and it is increasing (American Heart Association, 2007). The incidence in Hispanics and whites is about the same.

SUBJECTIVE DATA

1. Chest pain
2. Dyspnea
3. Orthopnea
4. Cough
5. Fatigue
6. Cyanosis or pallor
7. Edema
8. Nocturia
9. Past history (hypertension, elevated cholesterol, heart murmur, rheumatic fever, anemia, heart disease)
10. Family history (hypertension, obesity, diabetes, coronary artery disease)
11. Lifestyle (diet high in cholesterol, calories, or salt; smoking; alcohol use; drugs; amount of exercise)

OBJECTIVE DATA

PREPARATION

To evaluate the carotid arteries, the person may be sitting up. To assess the jugular veins and the precordium, the person should be supine with the head and chest slightly elevated. Stand on the person's right side.

EQUIPMENT NEEDED

Marking pen
Small ruler marked in centimeters
Stethoscope with diaphragm and bell endpieces
Alcohol wipe (to clean endpiece)

Normal Range of Findings	Abnormal Findings

The Neck Vessels

Palpate the Carotid Artery

Gently palpate only one carotid artery at a time to avoid compromising arterial blood to the brain.

Feel the contour and amplitude of the pulse. Normally, the contour is smooth, with a rapid upstroke and slower downstroke, and the normal strength is 2+ or moderate (see Chapter 13) and equal bilaterally.

Diminished pulse feels small and weak and occurs with decreased stroke volume.

Increased pulse feels full and strong and occurs with hyperkinetic states (see Table 13–1, p. 151).

Auscultate the Carotid Artery

For persons older than middle age or who show symptoms or signs of cardiovascular disease, auscultate each carotid artery for the presence of a **bruit.** This is a blowing, swishing sound indicating blood flow turbulence; normally, there is none.

Keep the neck in a neutral position. Lightly apply the bell of the stethoscope over the carotid artery at three levels: (1) the angle of the jaw, (2) the midcervical area, and (3) the base of the neck. Avoid compressing the artery, because this could create an artificial bruit. Ask the person to hold his or her breath while you listen.

A **bruit** indicates turbulence due to a local vascular cause, e.g., atherosclerotic narrowing.

A carotid bruit is audible when the lumen is occluded by $\frac{1}{2}$ to $\frac{2}{3}$. Bruit loudness increases as the atherosclerosis worsens until the lumen is occluded by $\frac{2}{3}$. When the lumen is completely occluded, the bruit disappears. Thus, absence of a bruit is not a sure indication of absence of a carotid lesion.

A **murmur** sounds much the same but is caused by a cardiac disorder. Some aortic valve murmurs radiate to the neck and must be distinguished from a local bruit.

Inspect the Jugular Venous Pulse

Position the person supine with the torso elevated anywhere from a 30- to a 45-degree angle. Remove the pillow to avoid flexing the neck. Turn the person's head slightly away from the examined side, and direct a strong light tangentially onto the neck to highlight pulsations and shadows.

Note the external jugular veins overlying the sternomastoid muscle. In some persons, the veins are not visible at all; in others, they are full in the supine position. As the person is raised to a sitting position, these external jugulars flatten and disappear, usually at 45 degrees.

Unilateral distention of external jugular veins is due to local cause, e.g., kinking or aneurysm.

Fully distended external jugular veins above 45 degrees signify increased central venous pressure (CVP).

Normal Range of Findings	Abnormal Findings

The Precordium

Inspect the Anterior Chest

You may or may not see the **apical impulse**. When visible, it occupies the fourth or fifth intercostal space, at or inside the midclavicular line. It is easier to see in children or those with thin chest walls.

A **heave** or **lift** is a sustained forceful thrusting of the ventricle during systole. It occurs with ventricular hypertrophy and is seen at the sternal border or the apex.

Palpate the Apical Impulse

(This used to be called the point of maximal impulse, or PMI.)

Localize the apical impulse precisely using one finger pad.

Note:
- Location—The apical impulse should occupy only one interspace, the fourth or fifth, and be at or medial to the midclavicular line
- Size—Normally 1 cm × 2 cm
- Amplitude—Normally a short, gentle tap
- Duration—Short, normally occupies only first half of systole

The apical impulse is palpable in about half of adults. It is not palpable with obese persons or persons with thick chest walls. With high cardiac output states (anxiety, fever, hyperthyroidism, anemia), the apical impulse increases in amplitude and duration.

Cardiac enlargement:
- Left ventricular dilatation (volume overload) displaces apical impulse down and to the left and increases size more than one space.
- Increased force and duration but no change in location occurs with left ventricular hypertrophy and no dilatation (pressure overload).

Apical impulse is not palpable with pulmonary emphysema due to the hyperinflated lungs that override the heart.

Palpate Across the Precordium

Using the palmar aspects of your four fingers, gently palpate the apex, the left sternal border, and the base, searching for any other pulsations: normally there are none. If any are present, note the timing. Use the carotid artery pulsation as a guide or auscultate as you palpate.

A **thrill** is a palpable vibration. It feels like the throat of a purring cat. The thrill signifies turbulent blood flow and accompanies loud murmurs. Absence of a thrill, however, does not necessarily rule out the presence of a murmur.

Auscultate the Heart Sounds

Identify the auscultatory areas where you will listen. The four traditional valve "areas" (Fig. 12–5) are not over the actual anatomic locations of the

Normal Range of Findings	Abnormal Findings

12-5   Auscultatory areas.

valves but are the sites on the chest wall where sounds produced by the valves are best heard:

- Second right interspace—Aortic valve area
- Second left interspace—Pulmonic valve area
- Left lower sternal border—Tricuspid valve area
- Fifth interspace at around left midclavicular line—Mitral valve area

Do not limit your auscultation to only four locations, because sounds produced by the valves may be heard all over the precordium. Learn to inch your stethoscope in a Z-pattern, from the base of the heart across and down, then over to the apex; or, start at the apex and work your way up. Include the sites shown in Figure 12–5.

Normal Range of Findings	Abnormal Findings

Begin with the diaphragm end-piece and clean it using an alcohol wipe. Use the following routine: (1) Note the rate and rhythm; (2) identify S_1 and S_2; (3) assess S_1 and S_2 separately; (4) listen for extra heart sounds; and (5) listen for murmurs.

Note the Rate and Rhythm. The rate changes normally from 60 to 100 beats per minute. The rhythm should be regular, although **sinus arrhythmia** occurs normally in young adults and children. With sinus arrhythmia, the rhythm varies with the person's breathing, increasing at the peak of inspiration, and slowing with expiration. Note any other irregular rhythm.

Identify S_1 and S_2. Usually, you can identify S_1 instantly because you hear a pair of sounds close together ("lub-dup"), and S_1 is the first of the pair. Other guidelines to distinguish S_1 from S_2 are as follows:

- S_1 is louder than S_2 at the apex; S_2 is louder than S_1 at the base.
- S_1 coincides with the carotid artery pulsation (Fig. 12–6).
- S_1 coincides with the R wave (the upstroke of the QRS complex) if the person is on an ECG monitor.

Premature beat—An isolated beat is early or a pattern occurs in which every third or fourth beat sounds early.

Irregularly-irregular—No pattern to the sounds; beats come rapidly and at random intervals.

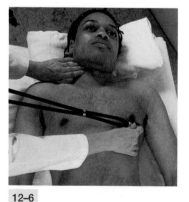

12–6

Normal Range of Findings	Abnormal Findings

Listen to S₁ and S₂ Separately. Note whether each heart sound is normal, accentuated, diminished, or split. Inch your diaphragm across the chest as you do this.

Causes of accentuated or diminished **S₁** (see Table 19–3, p. 515, in Jarvis: *Physical Examination and Health Assessment,* 5th ed.).

Both heart sounds are diminished with increased air or tissue between the heart and your stethoscope, such as emphysema (hyperinflated lungs), obesity, and pericardial fluid.

First Heart Sound (S₁). Caused by closure of the AV valves, **S₁** signals the beginning of systole. You can hear it over the entire precordium, though it is loudest at the apex (Fig. 12–7).

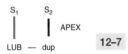

12–7

Second Heart Sound (S₂). **S₂** is associated with closure of the semilunar valves. You can hear it with the diaphragm over the entire precordium, although **S₂** is loudest at the base (Fig. 12–8).

Accentuated or diminished **S₂** (see Table 19–4, p. XXX, in Jarvis: *Physical Examination and Health Assessment,* 5th ed.).

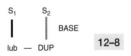

12–8

Splitting of S₂. A split **S₂** is a normal phenomenon that occurs toward the end of inspiration in some people. Recall that closure of the aortic and pulmonic valves is nearly synchronous. Because of the effects of respiration on the heart, inspiration separates the timing of the two valves' closure, and the aortic valve closes 0.06 second before the pulmonic valve. Instead of one "DUP," you hear a split sound—"T-DUP" (Fig. 12–9). During expiration, synchrony returns and the aortic and pulmonic components fuse together. A split **S₂** is heard only in the pulmonic valve area, the second left interspace.

Normal Range of Findings	Abnormal Findings

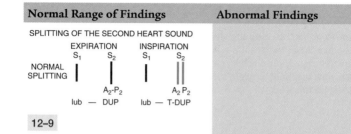

SPLITTING OF THE SECOND HEART SOUND

12–9

Concentrate on the split as you watch the person's chest rise up and down with breathing. The split S_2 occurs about every fourth heartbeat, fading in with inhalation and fading out with exhalation.

A *fixed split* is unaffected by respiration; the split is always there.

A *paradoxical split* is the opposite of what you would expect: The sounds fuse on inspiration and split on expiration (see Table 19–5, p. 516, in Jarvis: *Physical Examination and Health Assessment,* 5th ed.).

Focus on Systole, Then on Diastole, and Listen for Any *Extra Heart Sounds.* Listen with the diaphragm, then switch to the bell, covering all auscultatory areas. Usually, these are silent periods. When you do detect an extra heart sound, listen carefully to note its timing and characteristics.

During systole, the midsystolic click is the most common extra sound. The S_3 and S_4 occur in diastole; either may be normal or abnormal (see Table 12–1 on p. 148).

Listen for Murmurs. A murmur is a blowing, swooshing sound that occurs with turbulent blood flow in the heart or great vessels. Except for the innocent murmur described on the following page, murmurs are abnormal. If you hear a murmur, describe it by indicating these characteristics:

Timing. Systole or diastole.
Loudness. The intensity in terms of six grades:

Grade i—Barely audible, heard only in a quiet room and then with difficulty
Grade ii—Clearly audible, but faint
Grade iii—Moderately loud
Grade iv—Loud, associated with a thrill palpable on the chest wall

Conditions resulting in a murmur include (1) high rate of flow through a normal valve, such as with exercise, pregnancy, or thyrotoxicosis; (2) restricted forward blood flow through a stenotic valve; (3) backward flow through a regurgitant valve; and (4) blood flow through abnormal openings in the chambers.

For a description of pathologic murmurs, using these characteristics, see Table 19–10, p. 523, in Jarvis: *Physical Examination and Health Assessment,* 5th ed.

Normal Range of Findings	Abnormal Findings

Grade v—Very loud, heard with one edge of the stethoscope lifted off the chest wall

Grade vi—Loudest, still heard with entire stethoscope lifted just off the chest wall

Pitch. High, medium, or low.

Pattern. Growing louder (crescendo), tapering off (decrescendo), or increasing to a peak and then decreasing (crescendo-decrescendo, or diamond shaped). Since the entire murmur is just milliseconds long, it takes practice to diagnose pattern.

Quality. Musical, blowing, harsh, or rumbling.

Location. Area of maximum intensity of the murmur (where it is best heard) as noted by the valve area or intercostal spaces.

Radiation. Heard in another place on the precordium, the neck, the back, or the axilla.

Posture. Murmurs may disappear or be enhanced by a change in position.

Innocent Murmurs. Some murmurs are common in healthy children or adolescents and are termed **innocent** or **functional.** The contractile force of the heart is greater in children. This increases blood flow velocity. The increased velocity plus a smaller chest measurement makes an audible murmur.

The innocent murmur is generally soft (grade ii), midsystolic, short, crescendo-decrescendo, and with a vibratory or musical quality ("vooot" sound like fiddle strings). Also, the innocent murmur is heard at the second or third left intercostal space and disappears with sitting, and the young person has no associated signs of cardiac dysfunction.

Change Position. After auscultating in the supine position, roll the person toward his or her left side. Lis-

Although it is important to distinguish innocent murmurs from pathologic ones, it is best to suspect all murmurs as pathologic until proved otherwise. Diagnostic tests such as electrocardiography (ECG), ultrasonography, and echocardiography are needed to establish an accurate diagnosis.

S_3 and S_4 and the murmur of mitral stenosis may sometimes be heard only when on the left side.

Normal Range of Findings	Abnormal Findings
ten with the bell at the apex for the presence of any diastolic filling sounds. ♥ **DEVELOPMENTAL CARE** *Infants* Auscultate using the small (pediatric size) diaphragm and bell. The heart rate may range from 100 to 180 beats per minute immediately after birth, then stabilize to an average of 120 to 140 beats per minute. Infants normally have wide fluctuations with activity, from 170 beats per minute or more with crying or being active to 70 to 90 beats per minute with sleeping. Expect the heart rhythm to have sinus arrhythmia, the phasic speeding up or slowing down with the respiratory cycle. Rapid rates make it more challenging to evaluate heart sounds. Expect heart sounds to be louder in infants than in adults because of the infant's thinner chest wall. Splitting of S_2 just after the height of inspiration is common, not at birth but beginning a few hours after birth. Murmurs in the immediate newborn period do not necessarily indicate congenital heart disease. Murmurs are relatively common in the first 2 to 3 days because of fetal shunt closure. These murmurs are usually grade i or ii, systolic, accompany no other signs of cardiac disease, and disappear in 2 to 3 days. The murmur of patent ductus arteriosus (PDA) is a continuous machinery murmur, which disappears by 2 to 3 days. On the other hand, absence of a murmur in the immediate newborn period does not ensure a perfect heart; congenital defects can be present that are not signaled by an early	Persistent tachycardia: • >200 per minute in newborns or • >150 per minute in infants Bradycardia: • <90 per minute—All warrant further investigation Investigate any irregularity except sinus arrhythmia. Fixed split S_2 occurs with the murmur of atrial septal defect (ASD). Persistent murmur after 2 to 3 days, holosystolic murmurs, diastolic murmurs, and those that are loud all warrant further evaluation. For more information on murmurs due to congenital heart defects, see Table 19–9, p. 521, in Jarvis: *Physical Examination and Health Assessment,* 5th ed.

Normal Range of Findings	Abnormal Findings

murmur. It is best to listen frequently and to note and describe any murmur according to the characteristics listed on pp. 142–143.

Children
Note any extracardiac or cardiac signs that may indicate heart disease: normally, there are none.

Signs that indicate heart disease include poor weight gain, developmental delay, persistent tachycardia, tachypnea, dyspnea on exertion, cyanosis, and clubbing. Clubbing of fingers and toes does not appear until late in the first year, even with severe cyanotic defects.

The apical impulse is sometimes visible in children with thin chest walls.

Palpate the apical impulse: in the fourth intercostal space to the left of the midclavicular line until age 4; at the fourth interspace at the midclavicular line from age 4 to 6; and in the fifth interspace to the right of the midclavicular line at age 7.

Note any obvious bulge or any heave; these are not normal.

The apical impulse moves laterally with cardiac enlargement.
Thrill (a palpable vibration).

The average heart rate slows as the child grows older, although it is still variable with rest or activity.

The heart rhythm remains characterized by sinus arrhythmia. Physiologic S_3 is common in children (see Table 12–1). It occurs in early diastole, just after S_2, and is a dull, soft sound best heard at the apex.

Heart murmurs that are innocent (or functional) in origin are common through childhood. Most innocent murmurs have these characteristics: soft, relatively short, systolic ejection murmur; medium pitch; vibratory; and best heard at the left lower sternal or midsternal border, with no radiation to the apex, base, or back.

The Pregnant Female
The vital signs usually yield an increase in resting pulse rate of 10 to 15 beats per minute and a drop in blood pressure from the normal prepreg-

Normal Range of Findings	Abnormal Findings

nancy level. Blood pressure decreases to its lowest point during the second trimester and then slowly rises during the third trimester. Blood pressure varies with position. It is usually lowest in the left lateral recumbent position, a bit higher when supine (except for some who experience hypotension when supine), and highest when sitting.

Suspect pregnancy-induced hypertension with a sustained rise of 30 mm Hg systolic or 15 mm Hg diastolic under basal conditions.

Palpation of the apical impulse is higher and lateral as compared with the normal position, as the enlarging uterus elevates the diaphragm and displaces the heart up and to the left and rotates it on its long axis.

Auscultation of the heart sounds shows these changes due to the increased blood volume and workload:

Heart sounds
- Exaggerated splitting of S_1 and increased loudness of S_1
- A loud, easily heard S_3

Heart murmurs
- A systolic murmur in 90%, which disappears soon after delivery
- A soft, diastolic murmur heard transiently in 19%
- A continuous murmur arising from breast vasculature in 10%, the *mammary souffle* (pronounced soó fəl).

The Aging Adult

A gradual rise in systolic blood pressure is common with aging; the diastolic blood pressure stays fairly constant with a resulting widening of pulse pressure. Some older adults experience **orthostatic hypotension,** a sudden drop in blood pressure when rising to sit or stand.

The chest often increases in anteroposterior diameter with aging. This makes it more difficult to palpate the apical impulse and to hear the splitting of S_2. The S_4 often occurs

Normal Range of Findings	Abnormal Findings
in older people with no known cardiac disease. Occasional ectopic beats are common and do not necessarily indicate underlying heart disease. When in doubt, obtain an ECG; however, consider that the ECG records only one isolated minute and may need to be supplemented by 24-hour ambulatory heart monitoring.	

Summary Checklist

For a PDA-downloadable version go to http://evolve.elsevier.com/Jarvis.

Neck
1. **Carotid pulse:**
   Observe and palpate
2. **Observe jugular venous pulse**
3. **Estimate jugular venous pressure**

Precordium
1. **Inspection and palpation:**
   Describe location of apical impulse
   Note any heave (lift) or thrill
2. **Auscultation:**
   Identify anatomic areas where you listen
   Note rate and rhythm of heartbeat
   Identify S_1 and S_2, and note any variation
   Listen in systole and diastole for any extra heart sounds
   Listen in systole and diastole for any murmurs
   Repeat sequence with bell
   Listen at the apex with person in left lateral position

Nursing Diagnoses Commonly Associated with the Heart and Circulatory Disorders

Activity intolerance
Anxiety
Ineffective **Breathing** pattern
Decreased **Cardiac** output
Ineffective **Coping**
Fear
Complicated **Grieving**
Impaired **Home** maintenance
Risk for **Injury**

Sedentary **Lifestyle**
Noncompliance
Pain
Powerlessness
Ineffective **Role** performance
Self-care deficit
Ineffective **Sexuality** patterns
Ineffective **Tissue** perfusion

ABNORMAL FINDINGS

TABLE 12–1	Diastolic Extra Sounds

Third Heart Sound

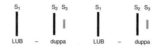

The S_3 is a ventricular filling sound. It occurs in early diastole during the rapid filling phase. Your hearing quickly accommodates to the S_3, so it is best heard when you listen initially. It sounds after S_2, is a dull soft sound, and is low pitched, like "distant thunder." It is heard best in a quiet room, at the apex, with the bell held tightly (just enough to form a seal), and with the person in the left lateral position.

The S_3 can be confused with a split S_2. Use these guidelines to distinguish the S_3:

- Location—The S_3 is heard at the apex or lower left sternal border; the split S_2 at the base.
- Respiratory variation—The S_3 does not vary in timing with respirations; the split S_2 does.
- Pitch—The S_3 is lower pitched; the pitch of the split S_2 stays the same.

The S_3 may be normal (physiologic) or abnormal (pathologic). The **physiologic S_3** is heard frequently in children and young adults; it occasionally may persist after age 40, especially in women. The normal S_3 usually disappears when the person sits up.

In adults, the S_3 is usually abnormal. The **pathologic S_3** is also called a **ventricular gallop** or an **S_3 gallop,** and it persists when sitting up. The S_3 indicates decreased compliance of the ventricles, as in congestive heart failure. The S_3 may be the earliest sign of heart failure.

The S_3 is also found in high cardiac output states in the absence of heart disease, such as hyperthyroidism, anemia, and pregnancy. When the primary conduction is corrected, the gallop disappears.

TABLE 12-1	Diastolic Extra Sounds—cont'd

Fourth Heart Sound

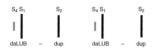

Pericardial Friction Rub

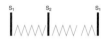

S_4 is a ventricular filling sound. It occurs when the atria contract late in diastole. It is heard immediately before S_1. This is a very soft sound, of very low pitch. You need a good bell, and you must listen for it. It is heard best at the apex, with the person in the left lateral position.

A **physiologic S_4** may occur in adults older than 40 or 50 with no evidence of cardiovascular disease, especially after exercise.

A **pathologic S_4** is termed an **atrial gallop** or an **S_4 gallop.** It occurs with decreased compliance of the ventricle, such as in coronary artery disease and cardiomyopathy, and with systolic overload (afterload), including outflow obstruction to the ventricle (aortic stenosis) and systemic hypertension.

Inflammation of the precordium gives rise to a **friction rub.** The sound is high pitched and scratchy, like sandpaper being rubbed. It is best heard with the diaphragm, with the person sitting up and leaning forward, and with the breath held in expiration.

A friction rub can be heard any place on the precordium but is usually best heard at the apex and left lower sternal border, places where the pericardium comes in close contact with the chest wall. Timing may be systolic and diastolic.

The friction rub of pericarditis is common during the first week after a myocardial infarction and may last only a few hours.

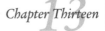
Peripheral Vascular System and Lymphatics

ANATOMY

The vascular system consists of the vessels in the body that transport fluid, such as blood or lymph.

The heart pumps freshly oxygenated blood and nutrients through the **arteries** to all body tissues. The major artery to the leg is the **femoral artery,** passing down under the inguinal ligament (Fig. 13–1).

Veins drain the deoxygenated blood and waste products from the tissues and return it to the heart (Fig. 13–2).

The **lymphatics** form a completely separate vessel system, which retrieves excess fluid and plasma proteins from the tissue spaces and returns them to the blood stream. The lymphatic system also forms a major part of the

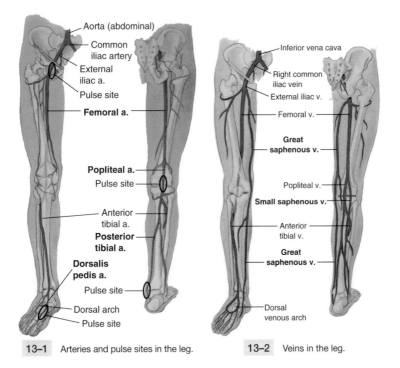

13–1 Arteries and pulse sites in the leg.

13–2 Veins in the leg.

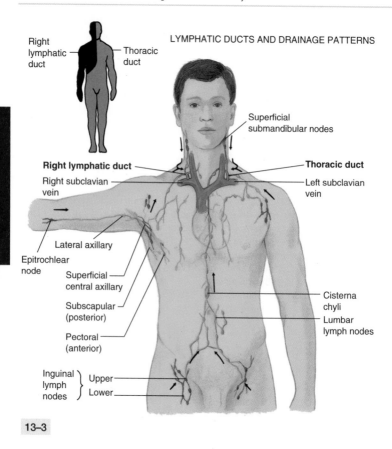

LYMPHATIC DUCTS AND DRAINAGE PATTERNS

Right lymphatic duct

Thoracic duct

Superficial submandibular nodes

Right lymphatic duct

Right subclavian vein

Thoracic duct

Left subclavian vein

Lateral axillary

Epitrochlear node

Superficial central axillary

Subscapular (posterior)

Pectoral (anterior)

Cisterna chyli

Lumbar lymph nodes

Inguinal lymph nodes { Upper
Lower

13–3

immune system that defends the body against disease.

Cervical lymph nodes drain the head and neck and are described in Chapter 6. Axillary lymph nodes drain the breast and upper arm and are described in Chapter 10.

The **epitrochlear** lymph node is in the antecubital fossa and drains the hand and lower arm (Fig. 13–3). The **inguinal** nodes in the groin drain most of the lymph of the lower extremity, the external genitalia, and the anterior abdominal wall.

SUBJECTIVE DATA

1. Leg pain or cramps
2. Skin changes on arms or legs
3. Swelling in legs
4. Lymph node enlargement (swollen glands)

OBJECTIVE DATA

PREPARATION

During a complete physical examination, examine the arms at the very beginning when you are checking the vital signs and the person is sitting. Examine the legs directly after the abdominal examination while the person is still supine. Then have the person stand up to evaluate the leg veins.

EQUIPMENT NEEDED (OCCASIONALLY)

Paper tape measure
Tourniquet or blood pressure cuff
Stethoscope
Doppler ultrasonic stethoscope

Normal Range of Findings	Abnormal Findings

Inspect and Palpate the Arms

Note color of **skin** and nail beds; temperature, texture, and turgor of skin; and the presence of any lesions, edema, or clubbing as described in Chapter 5.

Check **capillary refill.** Depress and blanch the nail beds; release and note the time for color return. Usually, the vessels refill within a fraction of a second. Consider it normal if the color returns in 1 or 2 seconds. Note conditions that can skew your findings, including a cool room, decreased body temperature, cigarette smoking, peripheral edema, and anemia.

Refill lasting more than 1 or 2 seconds signifies vasoconstriction or decreased cardiac output (hypovolemia, congestive heart failure, shock). The hands are cold, clammy, and pale.

The two arms should be **symmetric** in size.

Edema of upper extremities occurs when lymphatic drainage is obstructed, e.g., after breast surgery (see Table 20–2, p. 550, in Jarvis: *Physical Examination and Health Assessment,* 5th ed.).

Note the presence of any scars on hands and arms. Many occur normally with usual childhood abrasions or with occupations involving hand tools.

Needle tracks in antecubital fossae occur with intravenous drug use; linear scars in wrists may signify past self-inflicted injury.

Palpate both radial **pulses,** noting rate, rhythm, elasticity of vessel wall, and equal force. Grade the force (amplitude) on a three-point scale:

3+   increased, bounding
2+   **normal**
1+   weak
0   absent

Weak, thready pulse occurs with shock or peripheral arterial disease; full bounding pulse (3+) with hyperkinetic states (exercise, anxiety, fever), anemia, hyperthyroidism. Dropped beats; irregular pulse (see Table 13–1, pp. 159–160).

Normal Range of Findings	Abnormal Findings

Palpate the brachial pulses; their force should be equal bilaterally. Check the epitrochlear lymph node in the depression above and behind the medial condyle of the humerus.

An enlarged epitrochlear node occurs with infection of the hand or forearm.

Inspect and Palpate the Legs

Inspect both legs together, noting **skin** color, hair distribution, venous pattern, size (swelling or atrophy), and any skin lesions or ulcers.

Pallor with vasoconstriction; erythema with vasodilation; cyanosis.

Ulcers occur both with chronic arterial and chronic venous insufficiency (see Table 20–4, p. 552, in Jarvis: *Physical Examination and Health Assessment,* 5th ed.).

Hair normally covers the legs. Even if leg hair is shaved, you will still note hair on the dorsa of the toes.

Malnutrition: thin, shiny, atrophic skin, thick-ridged nails, loss of hair, ulcers, gangrene.
Malnutrition, pallor, and coolness occur with arterial insufficiency.

The **venous pattern** is normally flat and barely visible. Note obvious varicosities, although these are best assessed while the person is standing.

Both legs should be **symmetric in size** without swelling or atrophy. If the lower legs appear asymmetric, measure the calf circumference with a nonstretchable tape measure. Measure at the widest point, in exactly the same place, the same number of centimeters down from the patella or other landmark. Record your findings in centimeters.

Diffuse bilateral edema occurs with systemic illnesses, e.g., heart failure.
Unilateral swelling indicates a local obstruction, e.g., deep venous thrombosis, lymphedema.

Palpate for **temperature** along the legs and down to the feet, comparing symmetric spots. The skin should be warm and equal bilaterally. Bilateral cool feet may be due to environmental factors, such as cool room temperature, apprehension, and cigarette smoking. If there is any increase in temperature up the leg, note whether it is gradual or abrupt.

A unilateral cool foot or leg occurs with arterial deficit.

Palpate the **inguinal lymph nodes.** It is not unusual to find palpable nodes that are small (1 cm or less), movable, and nontender.

Enlarged nodes, tender or fixed in area.

Normal Range of Findings	Abnormal Findings

Palpate these **peripheral arteries** in both legs: femoral, popliteal, dorsalis pedis, and posterior tibial. Grade the force on the four-point scale.

Femoral Pulse. Locate the femoral arteries just below the inguinal ligament halfway between the pubis and anterior superior iliac spines (see Fig. 13–1). To help expose the femoral area, particularly in obese people, ask the person to bend his or her knees to the side in a froglike position. Press firmly and then slowly release, noting the pulse tap under your fingertips. If this pulse is weak or diminished, auscultate the site for a bruit.

Popliteal Pulse. This is a more diffuse pulse and can be difficult to localize. With the person's leg extended but relaxed, anchor your thumbs on the knee, and curl your fingers around into the fossa. Press your fingers forward hard to compress the artery against the bone. It is often just lateral to the medial tendon. A normal popliteal pulse is often impossible to palpate.

Posterior Tibial Pulse. Curve your fingers around the medial malleolus (Fig. 13–4). You will feel the tapping right behind it in the groove between the malleolus and the Achilles tendon.

Dorsalis Pedis Pulse. This requires a very light touch. It is normally just lateral to and parallel with the extensor tendon of the big toe (Fig. 13–5).

A bruit occurs with turbulent blood flow, indicating arterial occlusion.

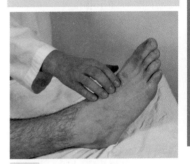

13–5   Dorsalis pedis pulse.

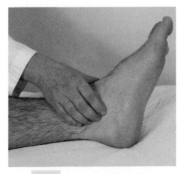

13–4   Posterior tibial pulse.

Normal Range of Findings	Abnormal Findings

Check for pretibial edema. Firmly depress the skin over the tibia or the medial malleolus for 5 seconds and release. Your finger should normally leave no indentation, although a pit is commonly seen if the person has been standing all day or during pregnancy. If pitting edema is present, grade it on this scale:

1+ Mild pitting, slight indentation, no perceptible swelling of the leg
2+ Moderate pitting, indentation subsides rapidly
3+ Deep pitting, indentation remains for a short time, leg looks swollen
4+ Very deep pitting, indentation lasts a long time, leg is very swollen

This scale is subjective.

Ask the person to stand so you can assess the venous system. Note any visible, dilated, or tortuous veins.

Additional Techniques

The Doppler Ultrasonic Stethoscope. Use this device to detect a weak peripheral pulse, to monitor blood pressure in infants and children, and to measure a low blood pressure or blood pressure in a lower extremity (Fig. 13–6).

Abnormal Findings:

Bilateral, dependent, pitting edema occurs with heart failure and hepatic cirrhosis.

Unilateral edema occurs with occlusion of a deep vein and unilaterally or bilaterally with lymphatic obstruction. With these factors, it is "brawny" or nonpitting and feels hard to the touch.

Varicosities occur in the saphenous veins (see Table 20–4, p. XXX, in Jarvis: *Physical Examination and Health Assessment,* 5th ed.).

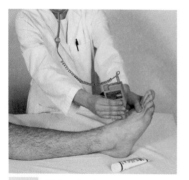

13–6   Using the Doppler to locate a pulse.

Normal Range of Findings	Abnormal Findings

The Doppler stethoscope magnifies pulsatile sounds from the heart and blood vessels. Place a drop of coupling gel on the end of the handheld transducer. Place the transducer over a pulse site, tilted at a 45-degree angle. Apply very light pressure; locate the pulse site by the swishing, whooshing sound.

✿ DEVELOPMENTAL CARE

Infants and Children

Transient acrocyanosis (i.e., symmetric cyanosis of the hands and wrists, feet and ankles) and skin mottling may occur at birth. Pulse force should be normal and symmetric. Pulse force should also be the same in the upper and lower extremities.

Weak pulses occur with vasoconstriction, diminished cardiac output.

Full, bounding pulses occur with patent ductus arteriosus due to left-to-right shunt.

Diminished or absent femoral pulses, while upper extremity pulses are normal, suggest coarctation of aorta.

Palpable lymph nodes occur often in normal infants and children. They are small, firm (shotty), mobile, and nontender. They may be the sequelae of past infection, e.g., inguinal nodes from a diaper rash or cervical nodes from a respiratory infection. Vaccinations can also produce local lymphadenopathy. Note characteristics of any palpable nodes and whether they are local or generalized.

Enlarged, warm, tender nodes indicate current infection. Look for source of infection.

The Pregnant Female

Expect diffuse, bilateral, pitting edema in the lower extremities, especially at the end of the day and into the third trimester. Varicose veins in the legs are also common in the third trimester.

The Aging Adult

The dorsalis pedis and posterior tibial pulses may become more difficult to find. Trophic changes associated with

Normal Range of Findings	Abnormal Findings
arterial insufficiency (thin, shiny skin; thick-ridged nails; loss of hair on lower legs) also occur normally with aging.	

Summary Checklist

For a PDA-downloadable version go to http://evolve.elsevier.com/Jarvis.

1. **Inspect arms:**
   Color and size
   Lesions
2. **Palpate pulses:**
   Radial
   Brachial
3. **Check epitrochlear node**
4. **Inspect legs:**
   Color and size
   Lesions
   Trophic skin changes

5. **Palpate temperature of feet and legs**
6. **Palpate inguinal nodes**
7. **Palpate pulses:**
   Femoral
   Popliteal
   Posterior tibial
   Dorsalis pedis

Nursing Diagnoses Commonly Associated with Peripheral Vascular System

Activity intolerance
Disturbed **Body** image
Fatigue
Risk for **Infection**
Insomnia
Impaired bed **Mobility**
Pain
Risk for **Peripheral** neurovascular
   dysfunction

Disturbed **Sensory** perception
   (tactile)
Sexual dysfunction
Disturbed **Sleep** pattern
Impaired **Tissue** integrity
Ineffective **Tissue** perfusion
   (peripheral)
Impaired **Walking**

ABNORMAL FINDINGS

TABLE 13–1	Variations in Arterial Pulse

Description	Associated With

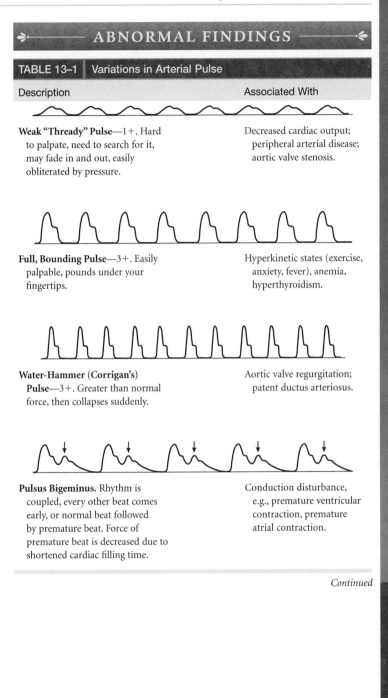

Weak "Thready" Pulse—1+. Hard to palpate, need to search for it, may fade in and out, easily obliterated by pressure.

Decreased cardiac output; peripheral arterial disease; aortic valve stenosis.

Full, Bounding Pulse—3+. Easily palpable, pounds under your fingertips.

Hyperkinetic states (exercise, anxiety, fever), anemia, hyperthyroidism.

Water-Hammer (Corrigan's) Pulse—3+. Greater than normal force, then collapses suddenly.

Aortic valve regurgitation; patent ductus arteriosus.

Pulsus Bigeminus. Rhythm is coupled, every other beat comes early, or normal beat followed by premature beat. Force of premature beat is decreased due to shortened cardiac filling time.

Conduction disturbance, e.g., premature ventricular contraction, premature atrial contraction.

Continued

TABLE 13–1 | Variations in Arterial Pulse—cont'd

Description	Associated With

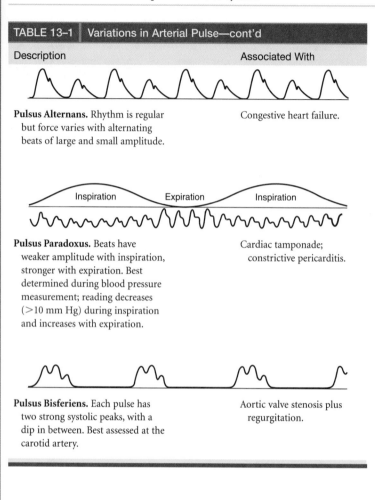

Pulsus Alternans. Rhythm is regular but force varies with alternating beats of large and small amplitude.

Congestive heart failure.

Pulsus Paradoxus. Beats have weaker amplitude with inspiration, stronger with expiration. Best determined during blood pressure measurement; reading decreases (>10 mm Hg) during inspiration and increases with expiration.

Cardiac tamponade; constrictive pericarditis.

Pulsus Bisferiens. Each pulse has two strong systolic peaks, with a dip in between. Best assessed at the carotid artery.

Aortic valve stenosis plus regurgitation.

Chapter Fourteen

Abdomen

The **abdomen** is a large oval cavity extending from the diaphragm down to the brim of the pelvis (Fig. 14–1). For convenience in description, the abdominal wall is divided into four quadrants by imaginary vertical and horizontal lines bisecting the umbilicus.

The **aorta** is just to the left of midline in the upper abdomen (Fig. 14–2).

At 2 cm below the umbilicus, it bifurcates into the right and left iliac arteries.

The bean-shaped **kidneys** are retroperitoneal, or posterior to the abdominal contents. The spleen is a soft mass of lymphatic tissue on the posterolateral wall of the abdomen just under the diaphragm.

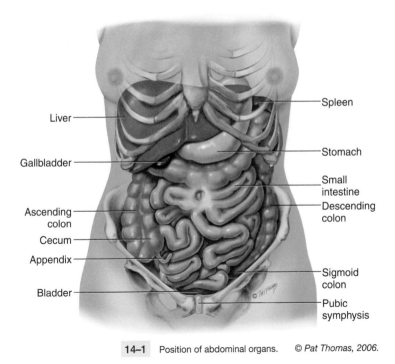

Liver

Gallbladder

Ascending colon

Cecum

Appendix

Bladder

Spleen

Stomach

Small intestine

Descending colon

Sigmoid colon

Pubic symphysis

14–1   Position of abdominal organs.   © *Pat Thomas, 2006.*

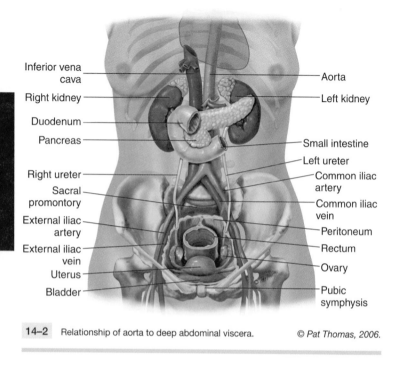

Inferior vena cava
Right kidney
Duodenum
Pancreas
Right ureter
Sacral promontory
External iliac artery
External iliac vein
Uterus
Bladder

Aorta
Left kidney
Small intestine
Left ureter
Common iliac artery
Common iliac vein
Peritoneum
Rectum
Ovary
Pubic symphysis

14–2 Relationship of aorta to deep abdominal viscera.   © Pat Thomas, 2006.

SUBJECTIVE DATA

1. Change in appetite
2. Dysphagia (difficulty swallowing)
3. Food intolerance
4. Abdominal pain
5. Nausea/vomiting
6. Bowel habits
7. Rectal conditions
8. Past abdominal history (ulcer, gallbladder disease, hepatitis, appendicitis, colitis, hernia)
9. Medications (prescription, over-the-counter, including antacids)
10. Alcohol, drug, cigarette use
11. Nutritional assessment (24-hour recall)

OBJECTIVE DATA

PREPARATION

Turn on a strong overhead light and a secondary stand light. Expose the abdomen so that it is fully visible. Drape the genitalia and female breasts.

The following measures will enhance abdominal wall relaxation:

- Have the person empty his or her bladder, saving a urine specimen if needed.
- Keep the room warm.
- Position the person supine, with the head on a pillow, knees bent or on a pillow, and the arms at the sides or across the chest.
- Keep the stethoscope endpiece warm, your hands warm, and your fingernails very short.
- Examine any painful areas last to avoid any muscle guarding.
- Use distraction: breathing exercises, emotive imagery, your low, soothing voice, and the person relating his or her abdominal history while you palpate.

EQUIPMENT NEEDED

Stethoscope
Small ruler marked in centimeters
Skin-marking pen
Alcohol wipe (to clean endpiece)

Normal Range of Findings	Abnormal Findings
Inspect Contour, Symmetry, Umbilicus, Skin, Pulsation or Movement, and Hair Distribution	
Contour. Stand on the person's right side and stoop to gaze across the abdomen. Determine the profile from the rib margin to the pubic bone, normally flat to rounded.	Protuberant abdomen, abdominal distention (see Table 21–1, pp. 588–589, in Jarvis: *Physical Examination and Health Assessment,* 5th ed.). Scaphoid abdomen occurs with malnourishment.
Symmetry. Shine a light across the abdomen toward you or shine it lengthwise across the person. The abdomen should be symmetric bilaterally. Note any localized bulging, visible mass, or asymmetry.	Bulges, masses. Hernia—Protrusion of abdominal viscera through abnormal opening in muscle wall (see Table 21–3, p. 591, in Jarvis: *Physical Examination and Health Assessment,* 5th ed.).
Umbilicus. It is normally midline and inverted with no sign of discoloration, inflammation, or hernia. It be-	Everted with ascites or underlying mass. Deeply sunken with obesity.

Normal Range of Findings	Abnormal Findings

comes everted and pushed upward with pregnancy.

Skin. The surface is smooth and even, with homogeneous color.

Enlarged and everted with umbilical hernia.

Redness with localized inflammation; jaundice with hepatitis (shows best in natural daylight).

Skin glistening and taut with ascites.

There are normally no lesions, although sometimes well-healed surgical scars are present. If a scar is present, draw its location in the person's record, indicating the length in centimeters.

Cutaneous angiomas (spider nevi) occur with portal hypertension or liver disease.

Lesions, rashes (see Chapter 5).

Pulsation or Movement. Pulsations from the aorta may show beneath the skin in the epigastric area, particularly in thin persons with good muscle wall relaxation. Respiratory movement also shows in the abdomen, particularly in males.

Marked pulsation of the aorta with widened pulse pressure (e.g., hypertension, aortic insufficiency, thyrotoxicosis), and aortic aneurysm.

Marked visible peristalsis, together with a distended abdomen, indicates intestinal obstruction.

Demeanor. A comfortable person is relaxed quietly on the examining table and has a benign facial expression and slow, even respirations.

Restlessness and constant turning to find comfort occur with the colicky pain of gastroenteritis or bowel obstruction.

Absolute stillness, resisting any movement, is demonstrated with the pain of peritonitis.

Knees flexed up, facial grimacing, and rapid, uneven respirations also indicate pain.

Auscultate Bowel Sounds and Vascular Sounds

This is done next because percussion and palpation can increase peristalsis, which would give a false interpretation of bowel sounds. Use the diaphragm endpiece and hold the stethoscope lightly against the skin. Begin in the RLQ, at the ileocecal valve area, because bowel sounds are normally always present here.

Bowel Sounds. Note the character and frequency, normally high-pitched, gurgling, cascading sounds, occurring irregularly anywhere from 5 to 30 times per minute. Do not bother to count them. Judge if they are normal, hypoactive, or hyperactive.

Two distinct patterns of abnormal bowel sounds may occur:

1. **Hyperactive sounds** are loud, high-pitched, rushing, tinkling sounds that signal increased motility. They occur with early mechanical bowel obstruction, gastroen-

Normal Range of Findings	Abnormal Findings

teritis, brisk diarrhea, laxative use, and subsiding paralytic ileus.

2. **Hypoactive or absent** sounds follow abdominal surgery or occur with inflammation of the peritoneum or from late bowel obstruction (see Table 21–4, p. 592, in Jarvis: *Physical Examination and Health Assessment,* 5th ed.).

Vascular Sounds. Note the presence of any vascular sounds or **bruits.** Using firmer pressure, listen over the aorta, renal arteries, iliac and femoral arteries, especially in people with hypertension (Fig. 14–3). Usually, there is no such sound.

Note location, pitch, and timing of a vascular sound.

A systolic bruit is a pulsatile, blowing sound and occurs with occlusion of an artery.

Venous hum and peritoneal friction rub are rare (see Table 21–5, p. 593, in Jarvis: *Physical Examination and Health Assessment,* 5th ed.).

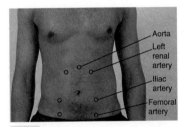

Aorta
Left renal artery
Iliac artery
Femoral artery

14–3 Sites to listen for vascular sounds.

Percuss General Tympany, Liver Span, and Splenic Dullness

General Tympany. Percuss lightly in all four quadrants. Tympany should predominate because air in the intestines rises to the surface when the person is supine.

Dullness occurs over a distended bladder, adipose tissue, fluid, or a mass.

Hyperresonance is present with gaseous distention.

Liver Span. Measure the height of the liver in the right midclavicular line. Begin in the area of lung resonance and percuss down the interspaces until the sound changes to a dull quality. Mark the spot, usually in the fifth intercostal space. Then find abdominal tympany and percuss up in the midclavicular line. Mark where the sound changes

Normal Range of Findings	Abnormal Findings

from tympany to a dull sound, normally at the right costal margin.

Measure the distance between the two marks; the normal liver span in the adult ranges from 6 to 12 cm (Fig. 14–4). Taller people have longer livers. Males also have a larger liver span than females of the same height. Overall, the mean liver span is 10.5 cm for males and 7 cm for females.

An enlarged liver span indicates liver enlargement or **hepatomegaly.**

Accurate detection of liver borders is confused by dullness above fifth intercostal space, which occurs with lung disease, e.g., pleural effusion or consolidation; lower border of dullness pushed up with ascites or pregnancy; gas distention in colon, which obscures lower border.

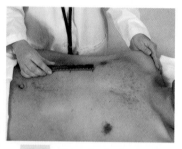

14–4 Measuring the liver span.

Splenic Dullness. Locate it by percussing a dull note from the 9th to 11th intercostal space just behind the left midaxillary line. The area of splenic dullness is normally not wider than 7 cm in adults and should not encroach on the normal tympany over the gastric air bubble.

A dull note forward of the midaxillary line indicates enlargement of the spleen, as occurs with mononucleosis, trauma, and infection.

Palpate Surface and Deep Areas, Liver Edge, Spleen, and Kidneys

Light and Deep Palpation. Begin with **light palpation.** With the first four fingers close together, depress the skin about 1 cm. Make a gentle rotary motion, lift the fingers (do not drag them), and move clockwise.

As you circle the abdomen, discriminate between voluntary muscle guarding and involuntary rigidity. Voluntary **guarding** occurs when the person is cold, tense, or ticklish. It is bilateral, and the muscles relax slightly during exhalation. Use relaxation

Muscle guarding.
Rigidity.
Large masses.
Tenderness.

Involuntary **rigidity** is a constant, boardlike hardness of the muscles. It is a protective mechanism accompanying acute inflammation of the peritoneum. It may be unilateral, and the same area usually becomes painful when the person increases

Normal Range of Findings

measures to try to eliminate this type of guarding, or it will interfere with deep palpation. If rigidity persists, it is probably involuntary.

Now perform **deep palpation,** pushing down about 5 to 8 cm (2 to 3 inches). Moving clockwise, explore the entire abdomen.

To overcome the resistance of a very large or obese abdomen, use a bimanual technique. Place your two hands on top of each other. The top hand does the pushing; the bottom hand is relaxed and can concentrate on the sense of palpation. With either technique, note the location, size, consistency, and mobility of any palpable organs and the presence of any abnormal enlargement, tenderness, or masses. Remember that some structures are normally palpable, as illustrated in Figure 14–5.

Abnormal Findings

intraabdominal pressure by attempting a sit-up.

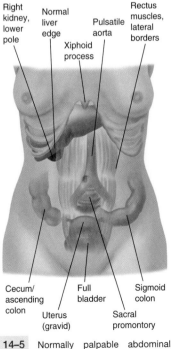

14–5   Normally palpable abdominal structures.

Normal Range of Findings	Abnormal Findings
There is normally mild tenderness when palpating the sigmoid colon. Any other tenderness should be investigated.	Tenderness occurs with local inflammation, with inflammation of the peritoneum or underlying organ, and with an enlarged organ whose capsule is stretched.

If you identify a mass, first distinguish it from a normally palpable structure or an enlarged organ. Then note its:
1. Location
2. Size
3. Shape
4. Consistency (soft, firm, hard)
5. Surface (smooth, nodular)
6. Mobility (including movement with respirations)
7. Pulsatility
8. Tenderness

Liver. Place your left hand under the person's back, parallel to the 11th and 12th ribs, and lift up to support the abdominal contents. Place your right hand on the RUQ, with fingers parallel to the midline (Fig. 14–6). Push deeply down and under the right costal margin. Ask the person to take a deep breath. It is normal to feel the edge of

Except with a depressed diaphragm, a liver palpated more than 1 to 2 cm below the right costal margin is considered enlarged. Record the number of centimeters it descends, and note its consistency (hard, nodular) and any tenderness.

The liver edge is often palpated below the right costal margin in people with chronic obstructive pulmonary disease (COPD), because their distended lungs and depressed diaphragm push the liver lower.

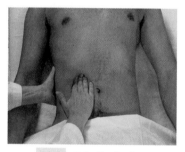

14–6   Palpating the liver.

the liver bump your fingertips as the diaphragm pushes it down during inhalation. It feels like a firm, regular ridge. The liver is often not palpable, and you may feel nothing firm.

Normal Range of Findings	Abnormal Findings

Spleen. Normally, the spleen is not palpable and must be enlarged three times its normal size to be felt. Reach your left hand over the abdomen and behind the left side at the 11th and 12th ribs. Lift up for support. Place your right hand obliquely on the LUQ with the fingers pointing toward the left axilla and just inferior to the rib margin. Push your hand deeply down and under the left costal margin, and ask the person to take a deep breath. You should feel nothing firm. When enlarged, the spleen slides out and bumps your fingertips.

The spleen enlarges with mononucleosis and trauma (see Table 21–6, p. 594, in Jarvis: *Physical Examination and Health Assessment,* 5th ed.). Refer the person with an enlarged spleen; do not continue to palpate. An enlarged spleen is friable and can rupture easily with overpalpation.

Describe the number of centimeters it extends below the left costal margin.

Kidneys. Search for the right kidney by placing your hands together in a "duckbill" position at the person's right flank. Press your two hands firmly, and ask the person to take a deep breath. With most people, you will feel no change. Occasionally, you may feel the lower pole of the right kidney as a round, smooth mass slide between your fingers. Either condition is normal.

The left kidney sits 1 cm higher than the right kidney and is not normally palpable.

Enlarged kidney.
Kidney mass.

Aorta. Using your opposing thumb and fingers, palpate the aortic pulsation in the upper abdomen slightly to the left of midline. It is normally 2.5 to 4 cm wide in adults, and pulsates in an anterior direction.

Widened aorta with aneurysm.
Prominent lateral pulsation with aortic aneurysm (see Table 21–6, p. 594, in Jarvis: *Physical Examination and Health Assessment,* 5th ed.).

Costovertebral Angle Tenderness. Place one hand over the 12th rib at the costovertebral angle on the back. Thump that hand with the ulnar edge of your other fist. The person normally feels a thud but no pain.

Sharp pain occurs with inflammation of the kidney or paranephric area.

Special Procedures

Rebound Tenderness. Choose a site away from the painful area. Hold your hand 90 degrees or perpendicu-

Normal Range of Findings	Abnormal Findings

lar to the abdomen. Push down slowly and deeply; then lift up *quickly*. This makes structures that are indented by palpation rebound suddenly. A normal, or negative, response is absence of pain on release of pressure. Perform this test at the end of the examination because it can cause severe pain and muscle rigidity.

Pain on release of pressure confirms rebound tenderness, which is a reliable sign of peritoneal inflammation.

Fluid Wave for Ascites. Place the ulnar edge of another examiner's hand or the patient's own hand firmly on the abdomen midline (Fig. 14–7). Place your left hand on the person's right flank. With your right hand, reach across the abdomen and give the left flank a firm strike. If ascites is present, the blow will generate a fluid

Ascites occurs with heart failure, portal hypertension, cirrhosis, hepatitis, pancreatitis, and cancer.

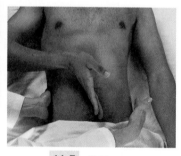

14–7   Fluid wave.

wave through the abdomen and you will feel a distinct tap on your left hand. If the abdomen is distended from gas or adipose tissue, you will feel no change.

A positive fluid wave test occurs with large amounts of ascitic fluid.

⚜ DEVELOPMENTAL CARE

The Infant

The contour of the abdomen is protuberant because of the immature abdominal musculature. The skin contains a fine, superficial venous

Scaphoid shape occurs with dehydration or malnutrition.
Dilated veins.

Normal Range of Findings	Abnormal Findings

pattern. This may be visible in children until puberty.

The abdomen shows respiratory movement. The only other abdominal movement is occasional peristalsis, which may be visible because of the thin musculature.

Auscultation yields only bowel sounds, the metallic tinkling of peristalsis. There should be no vascular sounds.

Marked peristalsis occurs with pyloric stenosis.

Bruit indicates stenosis or obstruction.

The Child

Under age 4 years, the abdomen looks protuberant when the child is both supine and standing. After age 4 years, the potbelly remains when standing because of lumbar lordosis, but the abdomen looks flat when supine. Normal movement on the abdomen includes respirations, which remain abdominal until 7 years of age.

A scaphoid abdomen is associated with dehydration or malnutrition.

Under 7 years of age, the absence of abdominal respirations occurs with inflammation of the peritoneum.

The Aging Adult

On inspection, you may note increased deposits of subcutaneous fat on the abdomen and hips as it is redistributed away from the extremities. The abdominal musculature is thinner and has less tone than that of the younger adult, so in the absence of obesity you may note peristalsis.

Because of the thinner, softer abdominal wall, the organs may be easier to palpate (in the absence of obesity). The liver is easier to palpate. Normally, you will feel the liver edge at or just below the costal margin. With distended lungs and a depressed diaphragm, the liver is palpated lower, descending 1 to 2 cm below the costal margin with inhalation. The kidneys are easier to palpate.

Abdominal rigidity with acute abdominal conditions is less common in aging persons.

With an acute abdomen, the aging person often complains of less pain than would a younger person.

Summary Checklist

For a PDA-downloadable version go to http://evolve.elsevier.com/Jarvis.

1. **Inspection:**
   Contour
   Symmetry
   Skin
   Pulsation or movement
   Demeanor
2. **Auscultation:**
   Bowel sounds
   Vascular sounds
3. **Percussion:**
   All four quadrants
   Borders of liver and spleen
4. **Palpation:**
   Light palpation in all four
   quadrants
   Deep palpation in all four
   quadrants
   Liver, spleen, kidneys

Nursing Diagnoses Commonly Associated with Abdominal Disorders

Constipation
Perceived **Constipation**
Diarrhea
Deficient **Fluid** volume
Bowel **Incontinence**
Functional **Incontinence**
Reflex **Incontinence**
Stress **Incontinence**
Total **Incontinence**
Urge **Incontinence**

Imbalanced **Nutrition:** less than body
requirements
Imbalanced **Nutrition:** more than
body requirements
Pain
Ineffective **Tissue** perfusion (renal
and gastrointestinal)
Urinary retention
Impaired **Urinary** elimination

Musculoskeletal System

The musculoskeletal system consists of the bones, joints, and muscles.

A **joint** (or articulation) is the place of union of two or more bones. Joints are the functional units of the musculoskeletal system because they permit the mobility needed for activities of daily living.

Synovial joints are freely movable because they have bones that are separated from each other and that are enclosed in a joint cavity (Fig. 15–1). This cavity is filled with a lubricant called synovial fluid.

In synovial joints, a layer of resilient **cartilage** covers the surface of opposing bones. The cartilage cushions the bones and gives a smooth surface to facilitate movement. The joint is surrounded by a fibrous capsule and is supported by ligaments. **Ligaments** are fibrous bands running directly from one bone to another that strengthen the joint and help prevent movement in undesirable directions. A **bursa** is an enclosed sac filled with viscous synovial fluid, much like a joint. Bursae are located in areas of potential friction (e.g., subacromial bursa of the shoulder, prepatellar bursa of the knee) and help muscles and tendons glide smoothly over bone.

Skeletal **muscle** is attached to bone by a **tendon**—a strong fibrous cord. Skeletal muscles produce the following movements (Fig. 15–2):

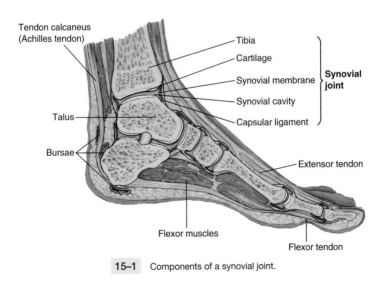

Tendon calcaneus
(Achilles tendon)

Tibia

Cartilage

Synovial membrane

Synovial cavity

Capsular ligament

Synovial joint

Talus

Bursae

Extensor tendon

Flexor muscles

Flexor tendon

15–1   Components of a synovial joint.

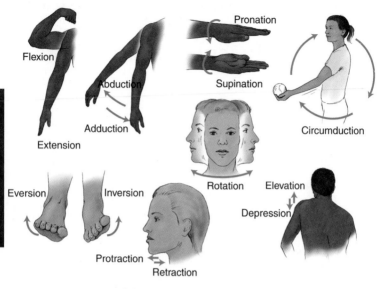

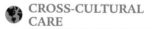

SKELETAL MUSCLE MOVEMENTS

15–2

© Pat Thomas, 2006.

1. Flexion—bending a limb at a joint
2. Extension—straightening a limb at a joint
3. Abduction—moving a limb away from the midline of the body
4. Adduction—moving a limb toward the midline of the body
5. Pronation—turning the forearm so the palm is down
6. Supination—turning the forearm so the palm is up
7. Circumduction—moving the arm in a circle around the shoulder
8. Inversion—moving the sole of the foot inward at the ankle
9. Eversion—moving the sole of the foot outward at the ankle
10. Rotation—moving the head around a central axis
11. Protraction—moving a body part forward and parallel to the ground
12. Retraction—moving a body part backward and parallel to the ground
13. Elevation—raising a body part
14. Depression—lowering a body part

CROSS-CULTURAL CARE

The long bones of blacks are significantly longer, narrower, and denser than those of whites (Overfield, 1995). Bone density measured by race and sex reveal that black males have the densest bones, thus accounting for the relatively low incidence of osteoporosis in this population. Bone density in the Chinese, Japanese, and Inuit is below that of white Americans (Overfield, 1995).

SUBJECTIVE DATA

1. Joints
   Pain
   Stiffness
   Swelling, heat
   Limitation of movement
2. Muscles
   Pain (cramps)
   Weakness
3. Bones
   Pain
   Deformity
   Trauma (fractures, sprains, dislocations)
4. Functional assessment (ADL)
   Any self-care deficit in bathing, toileting, dressing, grooming, eating, communicating, mobility
   Use of mobility aids
5. Self-care behaviors
   Occupational hazards
      Heavy lifting
      Repetitive motion to joints
   Nature of exercise program
   Recent weight gain

OBJECTIVE DATA

PREPARATION

The purpose of the musculoskeletal examination is to assess function for activities of daily living (ADL), as well as to screen for any abnormalities.

A **screening musculoskeletal examination** suffices for most people:

- Inspection and palpation of joints integrated with each body region
- Observation of ROM as person proceeds through motions necessary for an examination
- Age-specific screening measures, e.g., scoliosis screening for adolescents

A **complete musculoskeletal examination,** as described in this chapter, is appropriate for persons with articular disease, a history of musculoskeletal symptoms, or any problems with ADL.

EQUIPMENT NEEDED

Tape measure
Goniometer to measure joint angles
Skin-marking pen

Normal Range of Findings	Abnormal Findings
Order of the Examination	
Inspection	
Compare corresponding paired joints. Inspect for symmetry of structure and function as well as normal parameters for that joint.	

Normal Range of Findings	**Abnormal Findings**

Note the *size* and *contour* of the joint. Inspect the skin and tissues over the joints for *color, swelling,* and *masses* or *deformity.*

Presence of swelling is significant and signals joint irritation.

Palpation

Palpate each joint, including its skin, for temperature, its muscles, bony articulations, and area of joint capsule. Notice any heat, tenderness, swelling, and masses. Joints are normally not tender to palpation.

Heat, tenderness, and swelling signal inflammation.

Mass.

Range of Motion

Ask for **active** range of motion (ROM) while stabilizing the body area proximal to that being moved. Familiarize yourself with the type of each joint and its normal range of motion so you can recognize limitations.

If you see a limitation, gently attempt **passive** motion. Anchor the joint with one hand while your other hand slowly moves it to its limit. The normal ranges of active and passive motion should be the same.

If any limitation or increase in ROM occurs, use a **goniometer** to precisely measure the angles (Fig. 15–3). First extend the joint to neutral or 0 degrees. Center the 0 point of the goniometer on the joint. Keep the fixed arm of the goniometer on the 0 line and use the movable arm to measure; then flex the joint and measure through the goniometer to determine the angle of greatest flexion.

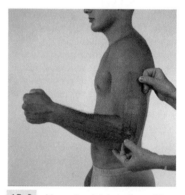

15–3   Measuring joint motion with a goniometer.

Joint motion normally causes no tenderness, pain, or crepitation. Do not confuse crepitation with the normal, discrete "crack" heard as a tendon or ligament slips over bone during motion, such as when you do a knee bend.

Crepitation is an audible and palpable crunching or grating that accompanies movement. Crepitation occurs when the articular surfaces in the joints are roughened, as with rheumatoid arthritis.

Muscle Testing

Test the strength of the prime mover muscle groups for each joint. Repeat the motions you elicited for active

Normal Range of Findings	Abnormal Findings

ROM. Ask the person to flex and hold as you apply opposing force. Muscle strength should be equal bilaterally and should fully resist your opposing force. (Note: Muscle status and joint status are interdependent and should be interpreted together. Chapter 16 discusses the examination of muscles for size and development, tone, and presence of tenderness.)

There is a wide variability of strength among people. You may wish to use a grading system from no voluntary movement to full strength, as shown in Table 15–1 on p. 191.

Cervical Spine

Inspect the alignment of head and neck. The spine should be straight and the head erect. **Palpate** the spinous processes and the sternomastoid, trapezius, and paravertebral muscles. They should feel firm, with no muscle spasm or tenderness.

Ask the person to follow these motions:*

Head tilted to one side.

Asymmetry of muscles. Tenderness.

Hard muscles with muscle spasm.

INSTRUCTIONS TO PERSON	MOTION AND EXPECTED RANGE
• Touch chin to chest.	Flexion of 45 degrees.
• Lift the chin toward the ceiling.	Hyperextension of 55 degrees.
• Touch each ear toward the corresponding shoulder. Do not lift up the shoulder.	Lateral bending of 40 degrees.
• Turn the chin toward each shoulder.	Rotation of 70 degrees.

Limited ROM.
Pain with movement.

Repeat the motions while applying opposing force. The person can normally maintain flexion against your full resistance. This also tests integrity of cranial nerve XI.

The person cannot hold flexion.

*DO NOT ATTEMPT IF YOU SUSPECT NECK TRAUMA.

Normal Range of Findings	Abnormal Findings

Upper Extremity

Shoulder

Inspect and compare both shoulders posteriorly and anteriorly. Check the size and contour of the joint and compare shoulders for equality of bony landmarks. There is normally no redness, muscular atrophy, deformity, or swelling.

Redness.
Inequality of bony landmarks.
Atrophy shows as lack of fullness (see Table 22–3, p. 644, in Jarvis: *Physical Examination and Health Assessment,* 5th ed.).

While standing in front of the person, **palpate** both shoulders, noting any muscular spasm or atrophy, swelling, heat, or tenderness.

Swelling.
Hard muscles with muscle spasm.

Test ROM by asking the person to perform four motions. Cup one hand over the shoulder during ROM to note any crepitation; normally there is none.

Tenderness or pain.

INSTRUCTIONS TO PERSON	MOTION AND EXPECTED RANGE	
1. With arms at sides and elbows extended, move both arms forward and up in wide vertical arcs. Then move them back.	Forward flexion of 180 degrees. Hyperextension up to 50 degrees.	Limited ROM. Asymmetry. Pain with motion. Crepitus with motion.
2. Rotate arms internally behind back, place back of hands as high as possible toward the scapulae.	Internal rotation of 90 degrees.	
3. With arms at sides and elbows extended, raise both arms in wide arcs in the coronal plane. Touch palms together above head.	Abduction of 180 degrees. Adduction of 50 degrees.	
4. Touch both hands behind the head, with elbows flexed and rotated posteriorly.	External rotation of 90 degrees.	

Test the **strength** of the shoulder muscles by asking the person to shrug

Normal Range of Findings	Abnormal Findings

the shoulders, flex forward and up, and abduct against your resistance. The shoulder shrug also tests the integrity of cranial nerve XI, the spinal accessory.

Elbow

Inspect the size and contour of the elbow in both flexed and extended positions. Look for any deformity, redness, or swelling.

Test ROM by asking the person to:

INSTRUCTIONS TO PERSON	MOTION AND EXPECTED RANGE
• Bend and straighten the elbow.	Flexion of 150 to 160 degrees, extension at 0. Some normal people lack 5 to 10 degrees of full extension, and others have 5 to 10 degrees of hyperextension.
• Hold the hand midway; then touch front and back sides of hand to table.	Movement of 90 degrees in pronation and supination.

While testing **muscle strength,** stabilize the person's arm with one hand (Fig. 15–4). Have the person

Swelling and redness (see Table 22–4, p. 645, in Jarvis: *Physical Examination and Health Assessment,* 5th ed.).

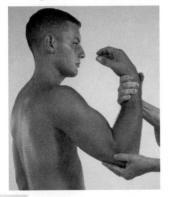

15–4 Stabilize the joint while testing muscle strength.

Normal Range of Findings	Abnormal Findings

flex the elbow against your resistance, applied just proximal to the wrist. Then ask the person to extend the elbow against your resistance.

Wrist and Hand

Inspect the hands and wrists on the dorsal and palmar sides, noting position, contour, and shape. The normal functional position of the hand shows the wrist in slight extension. This way the fingers can flex efficiently, and the thumb can oppose them for grip and manipulation. The fingers lie straight in the same axis as the forearm. There is normally no swelling or redness, deformity, or nodules.

Subluxation of wrist.
Ulnar deviation—fingers list to ulnar side.
Ankylosing—wrist in extreme flexion.

Dupuytren's contracture—flexion contracture of fingers.
Swan-neck or boutonnière deformity in fingers.

Hard nodules on fingers (see Table 22–5, pp. 646–648, in Jarvis: *Physical Examination and Health Assessment,* 5th ed.).

The skin looks smooth, with knuckle wrinkles present and no swelling or lesions. Muscles are full, with the palm showing a rounded mound proximal to the thumb (the *thenar eminence*), and a smaller rounded mound proximal to the little finger.

Atrophy of thenar eminence occurs with carpal tunnel syndrome as a result of compression of the median nerve.

Palpate each joint in the wrist and hands. Facing the person, support the hand with your fingers under it. Use gentle but firm pressure. Normally, the joint surfaces feel smooth, with no swelling, bogginess, nodules, or tenderness.

Ganglion in wrist.
Synovial swelling on dorsum.
Generalized swelling.
Tenderness.

Test ROM by using this procedure:

INSTRUCTIONS TO PERSON	MOTION AND EXPECTED RANGE
• Bend the hand up at the wrist.	Hyperextension of 70 degrees.
• Bend hand down at the wrist.	Palmar flexion of 90 degrees.
• Bend the fingers up and down at metacarpophalangeal joints.	Flexion of 90 degrees. Hyperextension of 30 degrees.

Loss of ROM here is the most common and the most significant type of functional loss of the wrist.
Limited motion.

Normal Range of Findings		Abnormal Findings
• With palms flat on table, turn them outward and in.	Ulnar deviation of 50 to 60 degrees, and radial deviation of 20 degrees.	Pain on movement.
• Spread fingers apart; make a fist.	Abduction of 20 degrees; fist tight. The responses should be equal bilaterally.	
• Touch the thumb to each finger and to the base of little finger.	The person is able to perform, and the responses are equal bilaterally.	

LOWER EXTREMITY

Hip

Wait to **inspect** the hip joint together with the spine a bit later in the examination as the person stands. At that time, note symmetric levels of iliac crests, gluteal folds, and equally sized buttocks. A smooth, even gait reflects equal leg lengths and functional hip motion.

Help the person into a supine position, and **palpate** the hip joints. The joints should feel stable and symmetric, with no tenderness or crepitation.

Pain with palpation.

Crepitation.

Assess **ROM** by asking the person to:

INSTRUCTIONS TO PERSON	MOTION AND EXPECTED RANGE	
• Raise each leg with knee extended.	Hip flexion of 90 degrees.	Limited motion. Pain with motion.
• Bend each knee up to the chest while keeping the other leg straight.	Hip flexion of 120 degrees. The opposite thigh should remain on the table.	Flexion flattens the lumbar spine; if this reveals a flexion deformity in the opposite hip, it is abnormal.

Normal Range of Findings		Abnormal Findings
• Flex knee and hip to 90 degrees. Stabilize by holding the thigh with one hand and the ankle with the other hand. Swing the foot outward. Swing the foot inward. (Foot and thigh move in opposing directions.)	Internal rotation of 40 degrees. External rotation of 45 degrees.	Limited internal rotation of hip is an early and reliable sign of hip disease.
• Swing leg laterally, then medially, with knee straight. Stabilize pelvis by pushing down on the opposite anterior superior iliac spine.	Abduction of 40 to 45 degrees; adduction of 20 to 30 degrees.	Limitation of abduction of the hip while supine is the most common motion dysfunction found in hip disease.
• When standing (later in examination), swing straight leg back behind body. Stabilize pelvis to eliminate exaggerated lumbar lordosis.	Hyperextension of 15 degrees when stabilized.	

Knee

The skin normally looks smooth, with even coloring and free of lesions.

Calluses.
Shiny and atrophic skin.
Inflammation.
Lesions, e.g., psoriasis.

Inspect lower leg alignment. The lower leg should extend in the same axis as the thigh.

Angulation deformity.
Flexion contracture.

Inspect the knee's shape and contour. Normally, there are distinct concavities, or hollows, on either side of the patella. Check them for any sign of fullness or swelling. Note other locations, such as the prepatellar bursa and the suprapatellar pouch, for any abnormal swelling.

Hollows disappear, then may bulge with synovial thickening or effusion (see Table 22–6, p. 649, in Jarvis: *Physical Examination and Health Assessment,* 5th ed.).

Check the quadriceps muscle in the anterior thigh for any atrophy. Because it is the prime mover of knee extension, this muscle is important for joint stability during weight-bearing.

Atrophy occurs with disuse or chronic disorders. It first appears in the medial part of the muscle, although it is difficult to note because the vastus medialis is relatively small.

Normal Range of Findings	Abnormal Findings

Check **ROM** by asking the person to:

INSTRUCTIONS TO PERSON	MOTION AND EXPECTED RANGE	
• Bend each knee.	Flexion of 130 to 150 degrees.	Limited in ROM.
• Extend each knee.	A straight line of 0 degrees, in some persons; a hyperextension of 15 degrees in others.	Contracture. Pain with motion.
• Check knee ROM during ambulation.		Limp. Sudden locking—the person is unable to extend the knee fully. This usually occurs with a painful and audible "pop" or "click." Sudden buckling, or "giving way," occurs with ligament injury, which causes weakness and instability.

Check muscle **strength** by asking the person to maintain knee flexion while you oppose by trying to pull the leg forward. Muscle extension is demonstrated by the person's success in rising from a seated position in a low chair or by rising from a squat without using the hands for support.

Ankle and Foot

Inspect and compare both feet, noting position of feet and toes, contour of joints, and skin characteristics. The foot should align with the long axis of the lower leg.

The toes point straight forward and lie flat. The ankles (malleoli) are smooth, bony prominences. The skin is normally smooth, with even coloring and no lesions. Note the locations of any calluses or bursal reactions because they reveal areas of abnormal friction. Examining well-worn shoes helps assess areas of wear and accommodation.

Hallux valgus and bunion.
Hammer toes.

Swelling or inflammation.

Calluses.
Ulcers.
(See Table 22–7, p. 650, in Jarvis: *Physical Examination and Health Assessment,* 5th ed.).

Normal Range of Findings	Abnormal Findings

Test **ROM** by asking the person to:

INSTRUCTIONS TO PERSON	MOTION AND EXPECTED RANGE
• Point toes toward the floor.	Plantar flexion of 45 degrees.
• Point toes toward your nose.	Dorsiflexion of 20 degrees.
• Turn soles of feet out, then in. (Stabilize the ankle with one hand, hold heel with the other to test the subtalar joint.)	Eversion of 20 degrees. Inversion of 30 degrees.
• Flex and straighten toes.	

Limited ROM.

Pain with motion.

Assess muscle **strength** by asking the person to maintain dorsiflexion and plantar flexion against your resistance.

Unable to hold flexion.

Spine

The person should be standing, draped in a gown open at the back. Place yourself far enough back so that you can see the entire back. Note if the spine is straight by following an imaginary vertical line from the head through the spinous processes and down through the gluteal cleft, and by noting equal horizontal positions for the shoulders, scapulae, iliac crests, and gluteal folds, and equal spaces between arm and lateral thorax on the two sides (Fig. 15–5, *A*). The person's knees and feet should be aligned with the trunk and should be pointing forward.

A difference in shoulder elevation and in level of scapulae and iliac crests occurs with scoliosis (see Table 15–2 on p. 192).

From the side, note the normal convex thoracic curve and concave lumbar curve (see Fig. 15–5, *B*). An enhanced thoracic curve, or **kyphosis,** is common in aging people. A pronounced lumbar curve, or **lordosis,** is common in obese people (see Table 15–2 on pp. 191–192).

Lateral tilting and forward bending occur with a herniated nucleus pulposus.

Normal Range of Findings	Abnormal Findings

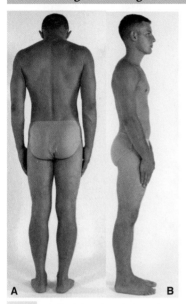

15–5 **A,** Straight spine. **B,** Normal curvature seen from side.

Check **ROM** of the spine by asking the person to bend forward and touch the toes. Look for flexion of 75 to 90 degrees and smoothness and symmetry of movement. Note that the concave lumbar curve should disappear with this motion, and the back should have a single, convex, C-shaped curve.

Stabilize the pelvis with your hands. Check ROM by asking the person to:

INSTRUCTIONS TO PERSON	MOTION AND EXPECTED RANGE	
• Bend sideways.	Lateral bending of 35 degrees.	Limited ROM.
• Bend backward.	Hyperextension of 30 degrees.	Pain with motion.
• Twist shoulders to one side, then the other.	Rotation of 30 degrees, bilaterally.	

Normal Range of Findings	Abnormal Findings

🔱 DEVELOPMENTAL CARE

Infants

Lift up the infant and examine the back. Note the normal, single, C-curve of the newborn's spine (Fig. 15–6). By 2 months of age, the infant can lift the head while prone. This builds the concave cervical spinal curve and indicates normal forearm strength.

Observe ROM through spontaneous movement of extremities.

Test muscle strength by lifting up the infant, with your hands under the baby's axillae. A baby with normal muscle strength wedges securely between your hands.

A baby who starts to slip between your hands shows weakness of the shoulder muscles.

Preschool and School-Age Children

Once the infant learns to crawl and then to walk, the waking hours show perpetual motion. This is convenient for your musculoskeletal assessment—you can observe the muscles and joints during spontaneous play before a table-top examination. Most young children enjoy showing off their physical accomplishments. For specific motions, coax the toddler: "Show me how you can walk to Mom," "Climb the stepstool." Ask the preschooler to hop on one foot or to jump.

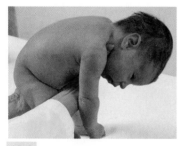

15–6   Normal spinal curvature in newborn.

Normal Range of Findings	Abnormal Findings

While the child is standing, note the posture. From behind, you should note a "plumb line" from the back of the head, along the spine, to the middle of the sacrum. Shoulders are level within 1 cm and scapulae are symmetric. From the side, lordosis is common throughout childhood, appearing more pronounced in children with a protuberant abdomen.

Lordosis is marked with muscular dystrophy and rickets.

Check the child's gait while walking away from and returning to you. Let the child wear socks, because a cold tile floor will distort the usual gait.

From 1 to 2 years of age, expect a broad-based gait, with arms out for balance. Weight-bearing falls on the inside of the foot. From 3 years of age, the base narrows and the arms are closer to the sides. Inspect the shoes for spots of greatest wear to aid your judgment of the gait. Normally, the shoes wear more on the outside of the heel and the inside of the toe.

Limp; usually caused by trauma, fatigue, or hip disease.

Adolescents

Proceed with the musculoskeletal examination you provide for the adult, except pay special note to spinal posture. Kyphosis is common during adolescence because of chronic poor posture.

Screen for **scoliosis** only when indicated (incidental finding or parental concern) (Fig. 15–7). Seat yourself behind the standing child, and ask the child to bend forward to touch the toes. Expect a straight vertical spine while standing and also while bending forward. Posterior ribs should be symmetric, with equal elevation of shoulders, scapulae, and iliac crests. You may wish to mark each spinous process with a felt marker when the adolescent bends forward. The line-up of ink dots when she or he stands up highlights even a subtle curve.

Be aware of the risk of sports-related injuries with the adolescent,

Scoliosis is exhibited as ribs hump up on one side as child bends forward and with unequal landmark elevation (see Table 15–2).

Normal Range of Findings	Abnormal Findings

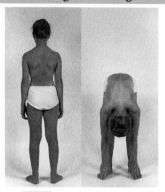

15-7   Scoliosis screening.

because sports participation and competition reach a height with this age group.

The Pregnant Female

Proceed through the examination described in the adult section. Expected postural changes in pregnancy include progressive lordosis and, toward the third trimester, anterior cervical flexion, kyphosis, and slumped shoulders (Fig. 15–8). When the pregnancy is at term, the protuberant abdomen and the relaxed mobility in the joints create the characteristic "waddling" gait.

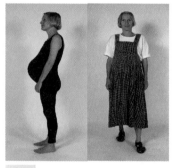

15-8

Normal Range of Findings	Abnormal Findings

The Aging Adult

Postural changes include a decrease in height, more apparent in the eighth and ninth decades (Fig. 15–9). "Lengthening of the arm–trunk axis" describes this shortening of the trunk with comparatively long extremities. Kyphosis is common, with a backward head tilt to compensate. This creates the outline of a figure 3 when you view this older adult from the left side. Slight flexion of hips and knees is also common.

Contour changes include a decrease of fat in the body periphery and fat deposition over the abdomen and hips. The bony prominences become more marked.

For most older adults, ROM testing proceeds as described earlier. ROM and muscle strength are much the same as with younger adults, provided there are no musculoskeletal illnesses or arthritic changes.

15–9 Postural changes with aging. (From Rossman I: *Clinical geriatrics,* ed 3, Philadelphia, 1986, Lippincott Williams and Wilkins.)

Functional Assessment

For those with advanced aging changes, arthritic changes, or musculoskeletal disability, perform a functional assessment for ADL. This applies the ROM and muscle strength assessments to the accomplishment of specific activities. You need to determine adequate and safe performance of functions essential for independent home life.

INSTRUCTIONS TO PERSON	COMMON ADAPTATION TO AGING CHANGES		
1. Walk (with shoes on).	Shuffling pattern; swaying; arms out to help balance; broader base of support; person may watch feet.	2. Climb up stairs.	Person holds hand rail; may haul body up with it; may lead with favored (stronger) leg.

INSTRUCTIONS TO PERSON	COMMON ADAPTATION TO AGING CHANGES		
3. Walk down stairs.	Holds handrail, sometimes with both hands. If the person is weak, he or she may descend sideways, lowering the weaker leg first. If the person is unsteady, he or she may watch feet.	5. Rise up from sitting in a chair.	Person uses arms to push off chair arms, upper trunk leans forward before body straightens, feet planted wide in broad base of support.
4. Pick up object from floor.	Person often bends at waist instead of bending knees; holds furniture to support while bending and straightening.	6. Rise up from lying in bed.	May roll to one side, push with arms to lift up torso, grab bedside table to increase leverage.

Summary Checklist

For a PDA-downloadable version go to http://evolve.elsevier.com/Jarvis.

For each joint to be examined:
1. **Inspection:**
   Size and contour of joint
   Skin color and characteristics
2. **Palpation of joint area:**
   Skin
   Muscles
   Bony articulations
   Joint capsule

3. **ROM:**
   Active
   Passive (if there is limitation in active ROM)
   Measure with goniometer (if there is abnormality in ROM)
4. **Muscle testing**

Nursing Diagnoses Commonly Associated with the Musculoskeletal Disorders

Activity intolerance
Disturbed **Body** image
Risk for **Disuse** syndrome
Deficient **Diversional** activity
Delayed **Growth** and development
Impaired **Home** maintenance management
Insomnia

Impaired Bed **Mobility**
Impaired Transfer **Mobility**
Impaired physical **Mobility**
Pain
Chronic **Pain**
Self-care deficit
Impaired **Skin** integrity
Risk for **Trauma**

ABNORMAL FINDINGS

TABLE 15–1	Grading Muscle Strength

Grade	Description	Percent Normal	Assessment
5	Full ROM against gravity, full resistance	100	Normal
4	Full ROM against gravity, some resistance	75	Good
3	Full ROM with gravity	50	Fair
2	Full ROM with gravity eliminated (passive motion)	25	Poor
1	Slight contraction	10	Trace
0	No contraction	0	Zero

TABLE 15–2	Curvatures of the Spine

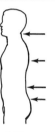
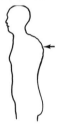

Normal Spinal Curvature

The vertebral column has four curves (a double-**S** shape). The cervical and lumbar curves are concave (inward), and the thoracic and sacrococcygeal curves are convex. The balanced or compensatory nature of these curves, together with the resilient intervertebral discs, allows the spine to absorb a great deal of shock.

Kyphosis

An exaggerated posterior curvature of the thoracic spine (humpback), associated with aging. Compensation may occur by hyperextension of head to maintain level of vision.

Continued

TABLE 15–2	Curvatures of the Spine—cont'd

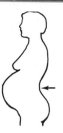

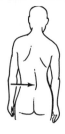

Lordosis

The normal lumbar concavity is further accentuated, associated with pregnancy, obesity, or kyphosis.

List

The spine tilts to one side, away from the affected side, usually associated with pressure on the local spinal nerve root from a herniated disc.

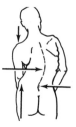

Scoliosis

A lateral S-shaped curvature of the thoracic and lumbar spine, usually with involved vertebrae rotation. Note rib hump on forward flexion. When standing, note unequal shoulder and scapular height, obvious curvature, unequal elbow level, unequal hip levels, and rib interspaces flared on convex side. More prevalent in adolescence, especially in girls.

Chapter Sixteen

Neurologic System

The nervous system can be divided into two parts—central and peripheral. The **central nervous system** (CNS) includes the brain and spinal cord. The **peripheral nervous system** includes the 12 pairs of cranial nerves, the 31 pairs of spinal nerves, and all their branches. The peripheral nervous system carries sensory messages *to* the CNS from sensory receptors and motor messages *from* the CNS out to muscles and glands, as well as autonomic messages that govern the internal organs and blood vessels.

THE CENTRAL NERVOUS SYSTEM

The **cerebral cortex** is the cerebrum's outer layer of nerve cell bodies, also called gray matter. The cerebral cortex is the center for humans' highest functions, governing thought, memory, reasoning, sensation, and voluntary movement (Fig. 16–1).

Each half of the cerebrum is a **hemisphere.** Each hemisphere is divided into four **lobes:** frontal, parietal, temporal, and occipital.

The lobes have certain areas that mediate specific functions as labeled

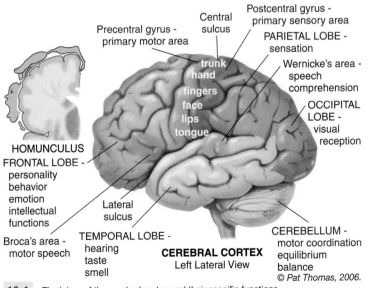

Precentral gyrus - primary motor area

Central sulcus

Postcentral gyrus - primary sensory area

PARIETAL LOBE - sensation

trunk
hand
fingers
face
lips
tongue

Wernicke's area - speech comprehension

OCCIPITAL LOBE - visual reception

HOMUNCULUS

FRONTAL LOBE - personality behavior emotion intellectual functions

Lateral sulcus

Broca's area - motor speech

TEMPORAL LOBE - hearing taste smell

CEREBRAL CORTEX Left Lateral View

CEREBELLUM - motor coordination equilibrium balance

© Pat Thomas, 2006.

16–1 The lobes of the cerebral cortex and their specific functions.

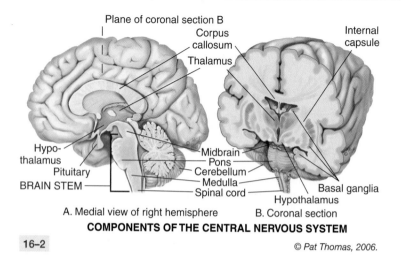

Plane of coronal section B

Corpus callosum

Thalamus

Internal capsule

Hypo-thalamus
Pituitary
BRAIN STEM

Midbrain
Pons
Cerebellum
Medulla
Spinal cord

Basal ganglia
Hypothalamus

A. Medial view of right hemisphere   B. Coronal section

COMPONENTS OF THE CENTRAL NERVOUS SYSTEM

16–2

© Pat Thomas, 2006.

in Figure 16–1. Damage to these specific cortical areas produces a corresponding loss of function: motor deficit, paralysis, loss of sensation, or impaired ability to understand and process language.

In addition to the cerebral cortex, the CNS has other vital components (Fig. 16–2).

The **thalamus** is the main relay station for incoming sensory pathways.

The **hypothalamus** controls temperature, sleep, emotions, autonomic activity, and the pituitary gland.

The **cerebellum** is concerned with motor coordination, equilibrium, and muscle tone.

The **midbrain** and **pons** contain motor neurons and motor and sensory tracts. The **medulla** contains fiber tracts and vital autonomic centers for respiration, heart, and gastrointestinal function.

The **spinal cord** is the main highway for ascending and descending fiber tracts that connect the brain to the spinal nerves, and it mediates reflexes.

THE PERIPHERAL NERVOUS SYSTEM

Cranial Nerves

Cranial nerves enter and exit the brain rather than the spinal cord (Fig. 16–3). The 12 pairs of cranial nerves supply primarily the head and neck, with the exception of the vagus nerve, which travels to the heart, respiratory muscles, stomach, and gallbladder.

Spinal Nerves

The 31 pairs of spinal nerves arise from the length of the spinal cord and supply the rest of the body (Fig. 16–4). They are named for the region of the spine from which they exit: 8 cervical, 12 thoracic, 5 lumbar, 5 sacral, and 1 coccygeal. They are "mixed" nerves because they contain both sensory and motor fibers.

A **dermatome** is a circumscribed skin area that is supplied mainly from one spinal cord segment through a particular spinal nerve.

I Olfactory	II Optic	III Oculomotor
		IV Trochlear
		VI Abducens

V Trigeminal

VII Facial

VIII Acoustic

IX Glossopharyngea

X Vagus

SENSORY
MOTOR

XII Hypoglossal

XI Spinal Accessory

CRANIAL NERVES

Cranial Nerve	Type	Function
I: Olfactory	Sensory	Smell
II: Optic	Sensory	Vision
III: Oculomotor	Mixed*	Motor—most EOM movement, opening of eyelids Parasympathetic—pupil constriction, lens shape
IV: Trochlear	Motor	Down and inward movement of eye
V: Trigeminal	Mixed	Motor—muscles of mastication Sensory—sensation of face and scalp, cornea, mucous membranes of mouth and nose
VI: Abducens	Motor	Lateral movement of eye
VII: Facial	Mixed	Motor—facial muscles, close eye, labial speech, close mouth Sensory—taste (sweet, salty, sour, bitter) on anterior two-thirds of tongue Parasympathetic—saliva and tear secretion
VIII: Acoustic	Sensory	Hearing and equilibrium
IX: Glosso-pharyngeal	Mixed	Motor—pharynx (phonation and swallowing) Sensory—taste on posterior one-third of tongue, pharynx (gag reflex) Parasympathetic—parotid gland, carotid reflex
X: Vagus	Mixed	Motor—pharynx and larynx (talking and swallowing) Sensory—general sensation from carotid body, carotid sinus, pharynx, viscera Parasympathetic—carotid reflex
XI: Spinal	Motor	Movement of trapezius and sternomastoid muscles
XII: Hypoglossal	Motor	Movement of tongue

*Mixed refers to a nerve carrying a combination of fibers: motor + sensory; motor + parasympathetic; or motor + sensory + parasympathetic.

16–3

Image © Pat Thomas, 2006.

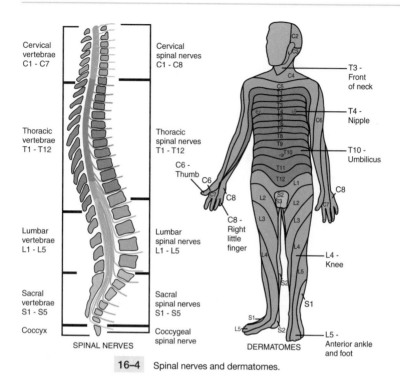

Cervical vertebrae
C1 - C7

Thoracic vertebrae
T1 - T12

Lumbar vertebrae
L1 - L5

Sacral vertebrae
S1 - S5

Coccyx

SPINAL NERVES

Cervical spinal nerves
C1 - C8

Thoracic spinal nerves
T1 - T12

C6 - Thumb

C8 - Right little finger

Lumbar spinal nerves
L1 - L5

Sacral spinal nerves
S1 - S5

Coccygeal spinal nerve

DERMATOMES

T3 - Front of neck

T4 - Nipple

T10 - Umbilicus

L4 - Knee

L5 - Anterior ankle and foot

16–4   Spinal nerves and dermatomes.

Reflex Arc

In the most simple reflex, the sensory afferent fibers carry the message from the receptor and travel through the dorsal root into the spinal cord (Fig. 16–5). They synapse in the cord with the motor neuron in the anterior horn. Motor efferent fibers leave via the ventral root and travel to the muscle.

The deep tendon or stretch reflex has five components:

1. An intact sensory nerve (afferent)
2. A functional synapse in the cord
3. An intact motor nerve fiber (efferent)
4. The neuromuscular junction
5. A competent muscle

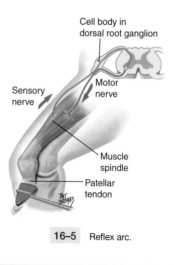

16–5   Reflex arc.

Cell body in dorsal root ganglion

Motor nerve

Sensory nerve

Muscle spindle

Patellar tendon

SUBJECTIVE DATA

1. Headache (unusually frequent or severe)
2. Head injury
3. Dizziness (feeling lightheaded or faint)/vertigo (feeling a rotational spinning)
4. Seizures
5. Tremors
6. Weakness or incoordination
7. Numbness or tingling
8. Difficulty swallowing
9. Difficulty speaking
10. Significant neurologic past history (brain attack, spinal cord injury, meningitis or encephalitis, congenital defect, alcoholism)

OBJECTIVE DATA

PREPARATION

Perform a **screening** neurologic examination (items identified in following sections) on seemingly well persons who have no significant subjective findings from the history.

Perform a **neurologic recheck** examination on persons with demonstrated neurologic deficits who require periodic assessments (e.g., hospitalized persons or those in extended care), using the examination sequence beginning on page 210.

EQUIPMENT NEEDED

Penlight
Tongue blade
Cotton swab
Cotton ball
Tuning fork (128 or 256 Hz)
Percussion hammer

Normal Range of Findings	Abnormal Findings
Mental Status Assess level of consciousness (see Chapter 2 and examination sequence on p. X).	
Test Selected Cranial Nerves Cranial Nerve II—Optic Nerve Test visual acuity and test visual fields by confrontation. When indicated, use the ophthalmoscope to examine the ocular fundus (see Chapter 7).	Visual field loss (see Table 14–5, p. 337, in Jarvis: *Physical Examination and Health Assessment,* 5th ed.). Papilledema with increased intracranial pressure; optic atrophy (see Table 14–9, p. 340, in Jarvis: *Physical Examination and Health Assessment,* 5th ed.).

Normal Range of Findings	Abnormal Findings

Cranial Nerves III, IV, and VI— Oculomotor, Trochlear, and Abducens Nerves

Palpebral fissures are usually equal in width or nearly so.

Ptosis (drooping) with myasthenia gravis, dysfunction of cranial nerve III, or Horner's syndrome (see Table 7–2 on p. 96).

Check pupils for size, regularity, equality, light reaction, and accommodation (see Chapter 7). The pupils are normally equal, round, react to light promptly, and react to accommodation (PERRLA).

Unequal size, constricted pupils, dilated pupils, or no response to light (see Table 7–3 on p. 78).

Assess extraocular movements by the cardinal positions of gaze (see Chapter 7).

Deviated gaze or limited movement.

Nystagmus is a back-and-forth oscillation of the eyes. End-point nystagmus, a few beats of horizontal nystagmus at extreme lateral gaze, occurs normally. Assess any other nystagmus carefully.

Cranial Nerve V—Trigeminal Nerve

Motor Function. Palpate the temporal and masseter muscles as the person clenches the teeth. Muscles should feel equally strong on both sides. Try to separate the jaws by pushing down on the chin; normally you cannot.

Decreased strength on one or both sides.

Pain with clenching of teeth.

Sensory Function. With the person's eyes closed, test light touch sensation by touching a cotton wisp to these designated areas on the person's face: forehead, cheeks, and chin. Ask the person to say "now" whenever the touch is felt.

Decreased or unequal sensation.

Cranial Nerve VII—Facial Nerve

Motor Function. Note mobility and facial symmetry as the person responds to these requests: smile, frown, close eyes tightly (against your attempt to open them), lift eyebrows, show teeth, and puff cheeks.

Muscle weakness is shown by loss of the nasolabial fold, drooping of one side of the face, lower eyelid sagging, and escape of air from only one puffed cheek when both are pressed in.

Normal Range of Findings	Abnormal Findings

Inspect and Palpate the Motor System

Muscles

Size. Muscle groups should be within the normal size limits for age and should be symmetric bilaterally. When muscles in the extremities appear asymmetric, measure each in centimeters and record the difference. A difference of 1 cm or less is not significant. Note that it is difficult to assess muscle mass in very obese people.

Atrophy—abnormally small muscle with a wasted appearance; occurs with disuse, injury, lower motor neuron disease, and muscle disease.

Hypertrophy—increased size and strength; occurs with isometric exercise.

Strength. Test homologous muscles simultaneously (see Chapter 15).

Cerebellar Function

Gait. Observe as the person walks 10 to 20 feet, turns, and returns to the starting point. Normally, the gait is smooth, rhythmic, and effortless; the opposing arm swing is coordinated; the turns are smooth. The step length is about 15 inches from heel to heel.

Stiff, immobile posture. Staggering or reeling. Wide base of support.

Lack of arm swing or rigid arms.

Unequal rhythm of steps. Slapping of foot. Scraping of toe of shoe.

Ask the person to walk a straight line in a heel-to-toe fashion (tandem walking) (Fig. 16–6). This decreases the base of support and accentuates any problem with coordination. Normally, the person can walk straight and stay balanced.

Ataxia—uncoordinated or unsteady gait.

Crooked line of walk.

Widens base to maintain balance.

Staggering, reeling, loss of balance.

An ataxia that did not appear with regular gait may now appear.

Swaying, falling, widening of base of feet to avoid falling.

Romberg Test. Ask the person to stand up with feet together and arms at the sides. Once in a stable position, ask the person to close the eyes and hold the position (Fig. 16–7). Wait about 20 seconds. Normally, a person can maintain posture and balance, although there may be slight swaying. (Stand close to catch the person in case he or she falls.)

Ask the person to perform a shallow knee bend or to hop in place, first on one leg, then the other. This

Positive Romberg sign is loss of balance increased by closing of the eyes. It occurs with cerebellar ataxia (multiple sclerosis, alcohol intoxication), loss of proprioception, and loss of vestibular function.

Normal Range of Findings	Abnormal Findings

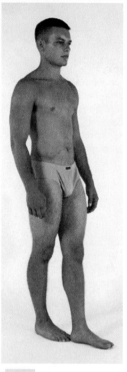

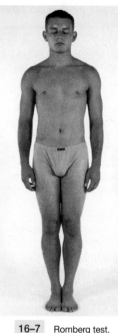

16-7   Romberg test.

16-6   Walk heel-to-toe.

demonstrates normal position sense, muscle strength, and cerebellar function. Note that some individuals cannot hop because of aging or obesity.

Assess the Sensory System

Make sure the person is alert, cooperative, and comfortable, and has an adequate attention span; otherwise, you may get misleading and invalid results. Testing of the sensory system can be fatiguing. You may need to repeat the examination later or break it into parts when the person tires.

Routine screening procedures include testing superficial pain, light

Normal Range of Findings	Abnormal Findings

touch, vibration in a few distal locations, and stereognosis.

The person's eyes should be closed during each test. Take time to explain what will be happening and exactly how you expect the person to respond.

Superficial Pain

Twist and break a tongue blade lengthwise, forming a sharp point at the fractured end and a dull spot at the rounded end. Lightly apply the sharp point and the dull end to the person's body in a random, unpredictable order (Fig. 16–8). Ask the person to say "sharp" or "dull," depending on the sensation felt. (Note that the sharp edge is used to test for pain; the dull edge is used as a general test of the person's responses.) Alternatively, break a cotton swab in half, forming a sharp point and using the dull spot at the cotton end.

Hypoalgesia—decreased pain sensation.

Analgesia—absent pain sensation.

Hyperalgesia—increased pain sensation.

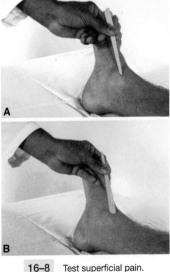

16–8   Test superficial pain.

Normal Range of Findings	Abnormal Findings
Let at least 2 seconds elapse between each stimulus to avoid *summation*. With summation, frequent consecutive stimuli are perceived as one strong stimulus.	

Light Touch

Apply a wisp of cotton to the skin. Stretch a cotton ball to make a long end and brush it over the skin in a random order of sites and at irregular intervals. Ask the person to say "now" or "yes" when touch is felt. Compare symmetric points.

Hypoesthesia—decreased touch sensation.
Anesthesia—absent touch sensation.
Hyperesthesia—increased touch sensation.

Vibration

Strike a low-pitch tuning fork on the heel of your hand and hold the base on a bony surface of the fingers and great toe. Ask the person to indicate when the vibration starts and stops. The normal response is vibration or a buzzing sensation on these distal areas. If no vibrations are felt, move proximally and test ulnar processes, ankles, patellae, and iliac crests. Compare the right side to the left. If you find a deficit, note whether it is gradual or abrupt.

Unable to feel vibration; states vibration stops when fork is still vibrating.
Loss of vibration sense occurs with peripheral neuropathy, e.g., diabetes and alcoholism. This is often the first sensation lost.

Stereognosis

Test the person's ability to recognize objects by feeling their forms, sizes, and weights. Place a familiar object (paper clip, key, coin) in the person's hand and ask the person to identify it with the eyes closed (Fig. 16–9). A person will normally explore it with the fingers and correctly name it. Test a different object in each hand; testing the left hand assesses right parietal lobe functioning.

Astereognosis—unable to identify object correctly; occurs in sensory cortex lesions.

Normal Range of Findings	Abnormal Findings

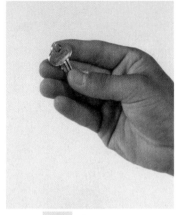

16-9   Stereognosis.

Test the Reflexes

Stretch or Deep Tendon Reflexes (DTRs)

For an adequate response, the limb should be relaxed and the muscle partially stretched. Stimulate the reflex by directing a short, snappy blow of the reflex hammer onto the muscle's insertion tendon. Strike a brief, well-aimed blow and bounce up promptly; do not let the hammer rest on the tendon. Use the pointed end of the reflex hammer when aiming at a smaller target (such as your thumb) on the tendon site; use the flat end when the target is wider or to diffuse the impact and prevent pain.

Use just enough force to get a response. Compare right and left sides; the responses should be equal. The reflex response is graded on a 4-point scale:

4 + Very brisk, hyperactive with clonus; indicative of disease
3 + Brisker than average; may indicate disease
2 + Average; normal
1 + Diminished; low normal
0   No response

Clonus is a set of short, jerking contractions of the same muscle.

Hyperreflexia is the exaggerated reflex seen when the monosynaptic reflex arc is released from the influence of higher cortical levels. This occurs with CNS upper motor

Normal Range of Findings	Abnormal Findings
	neuron lesions, e.g., after a brain attack (cerebrovascular accident).

Hyporeflexia, which is the absence of a reflex, is a lower motor neuron problem. It occurs with interruption of sensory afferents or destruction of motor efferents and anterior horn cells, e.g., spinal cord injury.

Biceps Reflex (C5 to C6). Support the person's forearm on yours; this position relaxes and partially flexes the person's arm. Place your thumb on the biceps tendon and strike a blow on your thumb. You can feel as well as see the normal response, which is flexion of the forearm (Fig. 16–10).

16–10   Biceps reflex.

Triceps Reflex (C7 to C8). Tell the person to let the arm "just go dead" as you suspend it by holding the upper arm. Strike the triceps tendon directly just above the elbow (Fig. 16–11). The normal response is extension of the forearm. Alternatively, hold the person's wrist across the chest to flex the arm at the elbow, and tap the tendon.

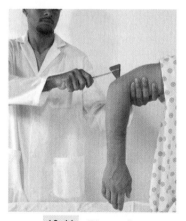

16–11   Triceps reflex.

Normal Range of Findings	Abnormal Findings

Patellar Reflex ("Knee Jerk") (L2 to L4). Let the lower legs dangle freely to flex the knee and stretch the tendons. Strike the tendon directly just below the patella (Fig. 16–12). Extension of the lower leg is the expected response. You also will palpate the contraction of the quadriceps.

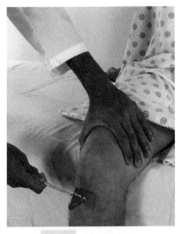

16–12   Patellar reflex.

Achilles Reflex ("Ankle Jerk") (L5 to S2). Position the person with the knee flexed and the hip externally rotated. Hold the foot in dorsiflexion and strike the Achilles tendon directly (Fig. 16–13). Feel the normal response as the foot plantar flexes against your hand.

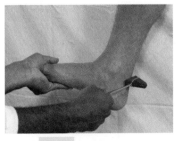

16–13   Achilles reflex.

Normal Range of Findings	Abnormal Findings
Plantar Reflex (L4 to S2). With the end of the reflex hammer, draw a light stroke up the lateral side of the sole of the foot and across the ball of the foot, like an upside-down **J** (Fig. 16–14, *A*). The normal response is plantar flexion of the toes and sometimes of the entire foot.	Except in infancy, the abnormal response is dorsiflexion of the big toe and fanning of all toes, which is a **positive Babinski sign.** This occurs with upper motor neuron disease of the pyramidal tract (see Fig. 16–14, B).

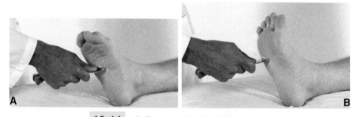

16–14   **A,** Plantar reflex. **B,** Babinski sign.

✿ DEVELOPMENTAL CARE

Infants (Birth to 12 Months)
Assessment includes noting that milestones you normally would expect for each month have indeed been achieved and that the early, more primitive reflexes are eliminated from the baby's repertory when they are supposed to be.

Observe spontaneous motor activity for smoothness and symmetry. Smoothness of movement suggests proper cerebellar function, as does the coordination involved in sucking and swallowing. To screen gross and fine motor coordination, use the Denver-II Developmental Screening test with its age-specific developmental milestones (see pp. 31–33 in Jarvis: *Physical Examination and Health Assessment,* 5th ed. for more information).

Check the muscle tone necessary for head control. With the baby supine and holding the wrists, pull the infant into a sitting position and note head control. The newborn will hold the head in almost the same plane as

Failure to attain a skill by expected time.

Persistence of reflex behavior beyond the normal time.

Delay in motor activity occurs with brain damage, mental retardation, peripheral neuromuscular damage, prolonged illness, and parental neglect.

Normal Range of Findings	Abnormal Findings

the body, and the head will balance briefly when the baby reaches a sitting position, then flop forward. (Even a premature infant shows some head flexion.) At 4 months of age, the head stays in line with the body and does not flop.

Because development progresses in a cephalocaudal direction, head lag is an early sign of brain damage.

After 6 months of age, any baby with failure to hold the head in midline when sitting should be referred.

Reflexes have a predictable time-table of appearance and departure. For the screening examination, check the rooting, grasp, Babinski, tonic neck, and Moro reflexes.

Rooting Reflex. Brush the infant's cheek near the mouth. The infant normally turns the head toward that side and opens the mouth. The reflex appears at birth and disappears within 3 or 4 months.

Palmar Grasp. Offer your finger and note tight grasp of all the baby's fingers. Sucking enhances grasp. You can often pull baby to a sit from grasp. The reflex is present at birth, is strongest at 1 to 2 months, and disappears at 3 to 4 months.

The reflex is absent with brain damage and with local muscle or nerve injury.
Persistence of the reflex after 4 months of age occurs with frontal lobe lesion.

Babinski Reflex. Stroke your finger up the lateral edge and across the ball of the infant's foot. Note fanning of toes (positive Babinski reflex; Fig. 16–15). The reflex is present at birth and disappears (changes to the adult response) by 24 months of age (variable).

Positive Babinski reflex after 2 or 2½ years of age occurs with pyramidal tract disease.

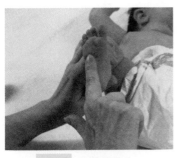

16–15   Babinski reflex.

Normal Range of Findings	Abnormal Findings

Tonic Neck Reflex. With the baby supine, relaxed, or sleeping, turn the head to one side with the chin over the shoulder. Note ipsilateral extension of the arm and leg and flexion of the opposite arm and leg; this is the "fencing" position. If you turn the infant's head to the opposite side, positions will reverse (Fig. 16–16). The reflex appears by 2 to 3 months, decreases at 3 to 4 months, and disappears by 4 to 6 months.

Persistence later in infancy occurs with brain damage.

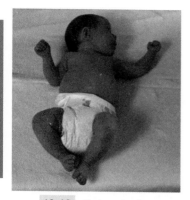

16–16   Tonic neck reflex.

Moro Reflex. Startle the infant by jarring the crib, making a loud noise, or supporting the head and back in a semisitting position and quickly lowering the infant to 30 degrees. The baby looks as if he or she is hugging a tree; that is, there is symmetric abduction and extension of the arms and legs, fanning fingers, and curling the index finger and thumb to C position. The infant then brings in both arms and legs (Fig. 16–17). The reflex is present at birth and disappears at 1 to 4 months.

Absence of the Moro reflex in the newborn or persistence after 5 months of age indicates severe CNS injury.

Absence of movement in one arm occurs with fracture of the humerus or clavicle and with brachial nerve palsy.

Absence in one leg occurs with a lower spinal cord problem or a dislocated hip.

A hyperactive Moro reflex occurs with tetany or CNS infection.

Normal Range of Findings	Abnormal Findings

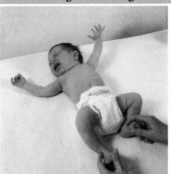

16–17   Moro reflex.

The Aging Adult

Use the same examination as used with younger adults. Be aware that some aging adults show a slower response to your requests, especially to those calling for coordination of movements.

Any decrease in muscle bulk is most apparent in the hand, as seen by guttering between the metacarpals. These dorsal hand muscles often look wasted, even with no apparent arthropathy. The grip strength remains relatively good.

Senile tremors occasionally occur. These benign tremors include an intention tremor of the hands, head nodding (as if saying yes or no), and tongue protrusion. There is no associated rigidity.

The gait may be slower, may be more deliberate, and may deviate slightly from a midline path compared with the gait in the younger person.

After 65 years of age, loss of the sensation of vibration at the ankle malleolus is common and is usually accompanied by loss of the ankle jerk. Tactile sensation may be impaired. The aging person may need stronger stimuli for light touch and especially pain.

Hand muscle atrophy is worsened with disuse and degenerative arthropathy.

Distinguish senile tremors from tremors of parkinsonism. The latter includes rigidity and slowness and weakness of voluntary movement.

Absence of a rhythmic, reciprocal gait pattern is seen in parkinsonism and hemiparesis.

Note any difference in sensation between the right and left sides, which may indicate a neurologic deficit.

Normal Range of Findings	Abnormal Findings

The deep tendon reflexes are less brisk. Those in the upper extremities are usually present, but the ankle jerks are commonly lost. Knee jerks may be lost, but this occurs less often.

The plantar reflex may be absent or difficult to interpret. Often you will not see a definite normal flexor response; however, you should still consider a definite extensor response to be abnormal.

Neurologic Recheck

Some hospitalized persons have head trauma or a neurologic deficit due to a systemic disease process. These people must be monitored closely for any improvement or deterioration in neurologic status and for any indication of increasing intracranial pressure.

Signs of increasing intracranial pressure signal impending cerebral disaster and death and require early and prompt intervention.

Use an abbreviation of the neurologic examination in the following sequence:
1. Level of consciousness
2. Motor function
3. Pupillary response
4. Vital signs

Level of Consciousness. A *change* in the level of consciousness is the single most important factor in this examination. It is the earliest and most sensitive index of change in neurologic status. Note the ease of *arousal* and the state of awareness, or *orientation*. Assess orientation by asking questions about:

A change in consciousness may be subtle. Note any decreasing level of consciousness, disorientation, memory loss, uncooperative behavior, or even complacency in a previously combative person.

Person—own name, occupation, names of workers around person, their occupation
Place—where person is, nature of building, city, state
Time—day of week, month, year

Vary the questions during repeat assessments so that the person is not merely memorizing answers. Note the

Normal Range of Findings	Abnormal Findings

quality and content of the verbal response, as well as articulation, fluency, manner of thinking, and any deficit in language comprehension or production (see Chapter 2, pp. 9–15).

A person is fully alert when his or her eyes open at your approach or spontaneously; when he or she is oriented to person, place, and time; and when he or she is able to follow verbal commands appropriately.

Review Table 2–1, Levels of Consciousness, Chapter 2, pp. 14-15.

If the person is not fully alert, increase the amount of stimulus used in this order:
1. Name called
2. Light touch on person's arm
3. Vigorous shake of shoulder
4. Pain applied (pinch nail bed, pinch trapezius muscle, rub your knuckles on the person's sternum)

Record the stimulus used as well as the person's response to it.

Motor Function. Check the voluntary movement of each extremity by giving the person specific commands. (This procedure also tests level of consciousness by noting the person's ability to follow commands.)

Ask the person to lift the eyebrows, frown, and bare the teeth. Note symmetric facial movements and bilateral nasolabial folds (cranial nerve VII).

Check upper arm strength by checking hand grasps. Ask the person to squeeze your fingers. Offer your two fingers, one on top of the other, so that a strong hand grasp does not hurt your knuckles.

Check lower extremities by asking the person to do straight leg raises. Ask the person to lift one leg at a time straight up off the bed. Full strength allows the leg to be lifted 90 degrees. If multiple trauma, pain, or equipment precludes this motion, ask the

Normal Range of Findings	Abnormal Findings

person to push one foot at a time against your hand's resistance, "like putting your foot on the gas pedal of your car."

For the person with decreased level of consciousness, note if movement occurs spontaneously, and as a result of noxious stimuli, such as pain or suctioning. An attempt to push away your hand after such stimuli is called *localizing* and characterized as purposeful movement.

Any abnormal posturing, decorticate rigidity, or decerebrate rigidity indicates diffuse brain injury (see Table 23–9, p. 711, in Jarvis: *Physical Examination and Health Assessment,* 5th ed.).

Pupillary Response. Note the size, shape, and symmetry of both pupils. Shine a light into each pupil and note the direct and consensual light reflex. Both pupils should constrict briskly. (Allow for the effects of any medication that could affect pupil size and reactivity.) When recording, pupil size is best expressed in millimeters. Tape a millimeter scale onto a tongue blade, and hold it next to the person's eyes for the most accurate measurement (Fig. 16–18).

In a brain-injured person, a sudden, unilateral, dilated, and nonreactive pupil is ominous. Cranial nerve III runs parallel to the brain stem. When increasing intracranial pressure pushes the brain stem down (uncal herniation), it puts pressure on cranial nerve III, causing pupil dilation.

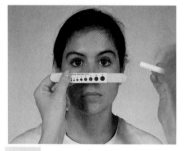

16–18   Measure pupil size in millimeters.

Vital Signs. Measure the temperature, pulse, respiration, and blood pressure as often as the person's condition warrants. Although they are vital to the overall assessment of the critically ill person, pulse and blood

Signs of increasing intracranial pressure, the *Cushing reflex:*

Normal Range of Findings	Abnormal Findings

pressure are notoriously unreliable parameters of CNS deficit. Any changes are late consequences of rising intracranial pressure.

The Glasgow Coma Scale (GCS). The GCS is an objective assessment that defines the level of consciousness by giving it a numeric value (Fig. 16–19).

Blood pressure—sudden elevation with widening pulse pressure

Pulse—decreased rate, slow and bounding

GLASGOW COMA SCALE		
BEST EYE OPENING RESPONSE (Record "C" if eyes closed by swelling)	Spontaneously	4
	To speech	3
	To pain	2
	No response	1
BEST MOTOR RESPONSE to painful stimuli (Record best upper limb response)	Obeys verbal command	6
	Localizes pain	5
	Flexion — withdrawal	4
	Flexion — abnormal*	3
	Extension — abnormal**	2
	No response	1
BEST VERBAL RESPONSE (Record "E" if endotracheal tube in place, "T" if tracheostomy tube in place)	Oriented × 3	5
	Conversation — confused	4
	Speech — inappropriate	3
	Sounds — incomprehensible	2
	No response	1
	* abnormal flexion — decorticate rigidity ** abnormal extension — decerebrate rigidity	

16–19

The scale is divided into three areas: eye opening, verbal response, and motor response. Each area is rated separately, and a number is given for the person's best response. The three numbers are added; the total score reflects the brain's functional level. A fully alert, normal person has a score of 15. Serial assessments can be plotted on a graph to illustrate visually whether the person is stable, improving, or deteriorating.

A score of 7 or less reflects coma.

Summary Checklist

For a PDA-downloadable version go to http://evolve.elsevier.com/Jarvis.

Neurologic Screening Examination
1. **Mental status (level of consciousness)**
2. **Cranial nerves:**
   II—optic
   III, IV, VI—extraocular muscles
   V—jaw muscles and facial sensation
   VII—facial mobility
3. **Motor function:**
   Gait and balance
   Knee flexion—hop or shallow knee bend

4. **Sensory function:**
   Superficial pain and light touch—arms and legs
   Vibration—arms and legs
   Stereognosis
5. **Reflexes:**
   Biceps
   Triceps
   Patellar
   Achilles
   Plantar

Nursing Diagnoses Commonly Associated with the Eyes and Visual Disorders

Activity intolerance
Anxiety
Risk for **Aspiration**
Risk for **Autonomic** dysreflexia
Risk for **Caregiver** role strain
Impaired verbal **Communication**
Risk for **Constipation**
Ineffective **Coping**
Deficient **Diversional** activity
Dysreflexia
Fear
Impaired **Home** maintenance
Hopelessness
Reflex urinary **Incontinence**
Total **Incontinence**

Impaired bed **Mobility**
Impaired physical **Mobility**
Unilateral **Neglect**
Disturbed **Sensory** perception (kinesthetic, tactile, visual)
Sexual dysfunction
Risk for impaired **Skin** integrity
Social isolation
Impaired **Swallowing**
Ineffective **Thermoregulation**
Disturbed **Thought** processes
Risk for **Trauma**
Impaired **Urinary** elimination
Impaired **Walking**

ABNORMAL FINDINGS

TABLE 16–1 | Abnormal Muscle Movement

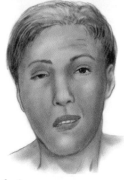

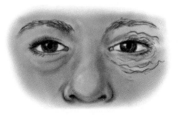

Paralysis

Decreased or loss of motor power due to problem with motor nerve or muscle fibers. Causes: acute—trauma, spinal cord injury, brain attack, poliomyelitis, polyneuritis, Bell's palsy; chronic—muscular dystrophy, diabetic neuropathy, multiple sclerosis; episodic—myasthenia gravis.

Fasciculation

Rapid, continuous twitching of resting muscle, that can be seen or palpated. Types: fine—occurs with lower motor neuron disease, associated with atrophy and weakness; coarse—occurs with cold exposure or fatigue and is not significant.

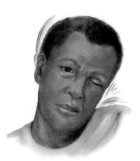

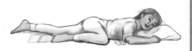

Tic

Involuntary, compulsive, repetitive twitching of a muscle group, e.g., wink, grimace, head movement, shoulder shrug; due to a neurologic cause, e.g., tardive dyskinesias, Tourette's syndrome, or psychogenic cause, e.g., habit tic.

Myoclonus

Rapid, sudden jerk at fairly regular intervals. A hiccup is a myoclonus of diaphragm. Single myoclonic arm or leg jerk is normal when the person is falling asleep; myoclonic jerks are severe with grand mal seizures.

TABLE 16–1   Abnormal Muscle Movement—(cont'd)

Tremor

Involuntary contraction of opposing muscle groups. Results in rhythmic, back-and-forth movement of one or more joints. May occur at rest or with voluntary movement. Tremors may be slow (3 to 6 per second) or rapid (10 to 20 per second).

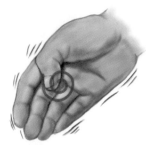 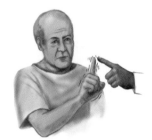

Rest Tremor	**Intention Tremor**
Coarse and slow (3 to 6 per second); partly or completely disappears with voluntary movement, e.g., "pill rolling" tremor of parkinsonism, with thumb and opposing fingers.	Rate varies; worse with voluntary movement. Occurs with cerebellar disease and multiple sclerosis. Essential tremor (familial)—a type of intention tremor; most common tremor with older people. Benign (no associated disease) but causes emotional stress.

Chapter Seventeen

Male Genitourinary System

ANATOMY

The **male genitalia** include the penis and scrotum externally, and the testis, epididymis and vas deferens internally (Fig. 17–1). The accessory glandular structures (prostate, seminal vesicles) are discussed in Chapter 19.

The **urethra** traverses the penis, and its meatus forms a slit at the glans tip.

The **scrotum** is a loose sac, which is a continuation of the abdominal wall. In each scrotal half is a **testis**, which produces sperm. The testis has a solid oval shape and is about 4 to 5 cm long by 3 cm wide in adults.

The testis is capped by the **epididymis,** which is a markedly coiled duct system that stores sperm. The epididymis is continuous with a muscular duct, the **vas deferens,** which approximates with other vessels to form the **spermatic cord.** The spermatic cord runs through the inguinal canal into the abdomen.

Puberty begins sometime between ages 9½ and 13½. The first sign is

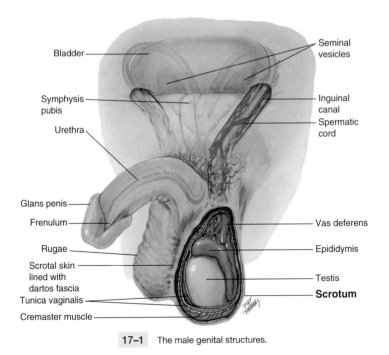

Bladder

Seminal vesicles

Symphysis pubis

Inguinal canal

Spermatic cord

Urethra

Glans penis

Frenulum

Vas deferens

Rugae

Epididymis

Scrotal skin lined with dartos fascia

Testis

Tunica vaginalis

Scrotum

Cremaster muscle

17–1   The male genital structures.

enlargement of the testes. Next, pubic hair appears, and then penis size increases. The stages of development are documented in Tanner's sexual maturity ratings (SMR).

The complete change in male genitalia development from preadolescent to adult takes around 3 years, although the normal range is 2 to 5 years.

SUBJECTIVE DATA

1. Frequency, urgency, and nocturia
2. Dysuria (pain or burning with urination)
3. Hesitancy and straining
4. Urine color (cloudy or hematuria)
5. Genitourinary history (kidney disease, kidney stones, flank pain, urinary tract infections, prostate trouble)
6. Penis—pain, lesion, discharge
7. Scrotum—pain, lumps
8. Self-care behaviors—perform testicular self-examination
9. Sexual activity and contraceptive use
10. Sexually transmitted disease (STD) contact

OBJECTIVE DATA

PREPARATION
Position the male standing with undershorts down and appropriate draping. The examiner should be sitting. Alternatively, the male may be supine for the first part of the examination and then stand during the hernia check.

EQUIPMENT NEEDED
Gloves—Wear gloves during every male genitalia examination
Glass slide for urethral specimen (occasionally)
Flashlight (occasionally)

Normal Range of Findings	Abnormal Findings
Inspect and Palpate the Penis The skin normally looks wrinkled, hairless, and without lesions.	Generalized swelling. Inflammation. Lesions: nodules, solitary ulcer (chancre), grouped vesicles or superficial ulcers, wartlike papules (see Table 24–3, p. 733, in Jarvis: *Physical Examination and Health Assessment,* 5th ed.).

Normal Range of Findings	Abnormal Findings
The glans looks smooth and without lesions. Ask the uncircumcised male to retract the foreskin or you retract it. It should move easily. After inspection, slide the foreskin back to the original position.	Phimosis—foreskin is advanced and fixed, so it cannot be retracted. Paraphimosis—foreskin is retracted and fixed, so it cannot be returned to original position.
The urethral meatus is positioned just about centrally on the glans.	Hypospadias—ventral location of meatus. Epispadias—dorsal location of meatus. (See Table 24–4, p. 735, in Jarvis: *Physical Examination and Health Assessment,* 5th ed.). Stricture—narrowed opening.
Compress the glans anteroposteriorly between your thumb and forefinger. The edge of the meatus should appear pink, smooth, and without discharge.	Edges that are red, everted, and edematous, along with purulent discharge, suggest urethritis (see Table 24–3, p. 734, in Jarvis: *Physical Examination and Health Assessment,* 5th ed.).
Palpate the shaft between your thumb and first two fingers. The penis normally feels smooth, semifirm, and nontender.	Nodule; induration. Tenderness.

Inspect and Palpate the Scrotum

Scrotal size varies with ambient room temperature. Asymmetry is normal, with the left scrotal half lower than the right. Lift the sac to inspect the posterior surface. Normally, there are no scrotal lesions except for the commonly found sebaceous cysts. These are yellowish, 1-cm nodules that are firm, nontender, and often multiple.	Scrotal swelling (edema) may be taut and pitting. This occurs with heart failure, renal failure, and local inflammation. Lesions. Inflammation.
Palpate each scrotal half between your thumb and first two fingers. Testes normally feel oval, firm and rubbery, and smooth and equal bilaterally. They are freely movable and slightly tender to moderate pressure. Each epididymis normally feels discrete, softer than the testis, smooth, and nontender.	Absent testis—may be a temporary migration or true cryptorchidism (see Table 24–5, p. 736, in Jarvis: *Physical Examination and Health Assessment,* 5th ed.). Atrophied testes—small and soft. Fixed testes. Nodules on testes or epididymides. Marked tenderness.

Normal Range of Findings	Abnormal Findings
Between your thumb and forefinger, palpate each spermatic cord along its length, from the epididymis up to the external inguinal ring. It should feel smooth and nontender.	Thickened cord. Soft, swollen, and tortuous cord—see varicocele, Table 24–5, p. 737, in Jarvis: *Physical Examination and Health Assessment,* 5th ed.
Normally, there are no other scrotal contents. If you do find a mass, note: • Is there any tenderness? • Is the mass distal or proximal to the testis? • Can you place your fingers over it? • Does it reduce when the person lies down? • Can you auscultate bowel sounds over it?	Abnormalities in the scrotum—hernia, tumor, orchitis, epididymitis, hydrocele, spermatocele, varicocele (see Table 24–5, pp. 737–738, in Jarvis: *Physical Examination and Health Assessment,* 5th ed.).

Inspect and Palpate for Hernia

Inspect the inguinal region for a bulge as the male stands and as he strains down. Normally, there is none.	Bulge at external inguinal ring or femoral canal. (A hernia may be present but easily reduced and appears only intermittently with an increase in intraabdominal pressure.)

Palpate the inguinal canal (Fig. 17–2). Ask the patient to shift his weight onto the unexamined leg. Place your index finger low on the scrotal half. Palpate up the length of

External inguinal ring

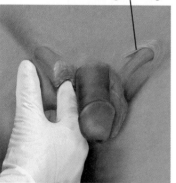

17–2   Palpate for inguinal hernia.

Normal Range of Findings	Abnormal Findings
the spermatic cord, invaginating the scrotal skin as you go, to the external inguinal ring. The inguinal ring feels like a triangular, slitlike opening, and it may or may not admit your finger. If it will admit your finger, gently insert it into the canal and ask the person to bear down. Normally, you will feel no change. Repeat the procedure on the other side. Palpate the femoral area for a bulge. Normally, you feel none.	Palpable herniating mass bumps your fingertip or pushes against the side of your finger (see Table 24–6, p. 739, in Jarvis: *Physical Examination and Health Assessment,* 5th ed.).

Inguinal Lymph Nodes

Palpate the horizontal chain along the groin inferior to the inguinal ligament and the vertical chain along the upper inner thigh. On occasion, it is normal to palpate an isolated node. It feels small (<1 cm), soft, discrete, and movable.	Enlarged, hard, matted, fixed nodes.

Testicular Self-Exam

Encourage self-care by instructing each male (from 13 to 14 years old through adulthood) in examining his own testicles every month.	The incidence of testicular cancer is not high, but testicular cancer most commonly occurs in young men ages 15 to 40.

A testicular tumor has no early symptoms. If it is detected early by palpation and treated, the prognosis is much improved. Early detection is enhanced if the person is familiar with the normal consistency of his testes. Phrase the teaching something like this:

A good time to examine the testicles is during the shower or bath when your hands and scrotum are warm. Cold hands stimulate a muscular (cremasteric) reflex, retracting the scrotal contents. The procedure is simple. Hold the scrotum in the palm of your hand, and gently feel each testicle using your thumb and first two fingers. If it hurts, you are using too much pressure. The testicle is egg

Normal Range of Findings	Abnormal Findings

shaped and movable. It feels rubbery with a smooth surface, like a hard-boiled egg. The epididymis is on top and behind the testicle; it feels a bit softer. If you notice a firm, painless lump, a hard area, or an overall enlarged testicle, call your physician for a further check.

🜨 DEVELOPMENTAL CARE

Infants and Children

Palpate the scrotum and testes. Take care not to elicit the cremasteric reflex that pulls the testes up into the inguinal canal. (1) Keep your hands warm and palpate from the external inguinal ring down. (2) Block the inguinal canals with the thumb and forefinger of your other hand to prevent the testes from retracting (Fig. 17–3).

Normally, the testes are descended and are equal in size bilaterally (1.5 to 2 cm until puberty). Once palpated, testes are considered descended, even if they have retracted momentarily at the next visit.

If the scrotal half feels empty, search for the testes along the inguinal canal and try to milk them down.

Cryptorchidism—undescended testes (those that have never descended). Undescended testes are common in premature infants. They occur in 3 to 4 percent of term infants, although most have descended by 3 months of age. The age at which a child should be referred differs among physicians (see Table 24–5, p. 736, in Jarvis: *Physical Examination and Health Assessment,* 5th ed.).

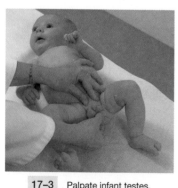

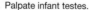
17–3 Palpate infant testes.

Normal Range of Findings	Abnormal Findings
Ask the toddler or child to squat with the knees flexed up: this pressure may force the testes down. Migratory testes (physiologic cryptorchidism) are common because of the strength of the cremasteric reflex and the small mass of the prepubertal testes. Note that the affected side has a normally developed scrotum and that the testis can be milked down. These testes descend at puberty and are normal. **The Aging Adult** In the older male, you may note thinner, graying pubic hair and a decreased size of the penis. The size of the testes may be decreased, and they may feel less firm. The scrotal sac is pendulous, with less rugae. The scrotal skin may become excoriated if the man continually sits on it.	With true cryptorchidism, the scrotum is atrophic.

Summary Checklist

For a PDA-downloadable version go to http://evolve.elsevier.com/Jarvis.

1. Inspect and palpate the penis
2. Inspect and palpate the scrotum
3. If a mass exists, note associated signs
4. Palpate for an inguinal hernia
5. Palpate the inguinal lymph nodes
6. Teach testicular self-examination

Nursing Diagnoses Commonly Associated with the Male Genitalia and Related Disorders

Anxiety
Delayed **Growth** and development
Incontinence
Pain
Rape trauma syndrome: compound reaction
Rape trauma syndrome: silent reaction

Sexual dysfunction
Ineffective **Sexuality** patterns
Impaired **Skin** integrity
Impaired **Urinary** elimination
Urinary retention

ABNORMAL FINDINGS

TABLE 17–1	Abnormalities in the Scrotum	
Disorder	Clinical Findings	Discussion
Absent Testis Cryptorchidism	S: Empty scrotal half O: Inspection—in true maldescent, atrophic scrotum on affected side Palpation—no testis A: Absent testis	True cryptorchidism—testes that have never descended. Incidence at birth is 3 to 4 percent, one-half of these descend in first month. Incidence with premature infants is 30 percent; in the adult 0.7 to 0.8 percent. True undescended testes have a histologic change by 6 years, causing decreased spermatogenesis and infertility.
Small Testis	S: (None) O: Palpation—small and soft (rarely may be firm) A: Small testis	Small and soft (<3.5 cm) indicates atrophy as with cirrhosis, hypopituitarism, following estrogen therapy, or as a sequelae of orchitis. Small and firm (<2 cm) occurs with Klinefelter's syndrome (hypogonadism).
Testicular Torsion	S: Excruciating pain in testicle of sudden onset, often during sleep or following trauma. May also have lower abdominal pain, nausea and vomiting, no fever O: Inspection—red, swollen scrotum, one testis (usually left) higher owing to rotation and shortening Palpation—cord feels thick, swollen, tender, epididymis may be anterior, cremasteric reflex is absent on side of torsion	Sudden twisting of spermatic cord. Occurs in late childhood, early adolescence, rare after age of 20 years. Torsion occurs usually on the left side. Faulty anchoring of testis on wall of scrotum allows testis to rotate. The anterior part of the testis rotates medially toward the other testis. Blood supply is cut off, resulting in ischemia and engorgement. This is an emergency requiring surgery; testis can become gangrenous in a few hours.

S = subjective data; O = objective data; A = assessment.
Illustrations © Pat Thomas, 2006.

TABLE 17–1	Abnormalities in the Scrotum—(cont'd)	
Disorder	Clinical Findings	Discussion
Epididymitis	S: Severe pain of sudden onset in scrotum, somewhat relieved by elevation (a positive Phren's sign); also rapid swelling, fever O: Inspection—enlarged scrotum; reddened Palpation—exquisitely tender; epididymis enlarged, indurated; may be hard to distinguish from testis. Overlying scrotal skin may be thick and edematous Laboratory—white blood cells and bacteria in urine A: Tender swelling of epididymis	Acute infection of epididymis commonly caused by prostatitis, after prostatectomy because of trauma of urethral instrumentation, or due to chlamydia, gonorrhea, or other bacterial infection. Often difficult to distinguish between epididymitis and testicular torsion.
Spermatic Cord Varicocele	S: Dull pain; constant pulling or dragging feeling; or may be asymptomatic O: Inspection—usually no sign. May show bluish color through light scrotal skin Palpation—when standing, feel soft, irregular mass posterior to and above testis; collapses when supine, refills when upright. Feels distinctive, like a "bag of worms" The testis on the side of the varicocele may be smaller owing to impaired circulation A: Soft mass on spermatic cord	A varicocele is dilated, tortuous varicose veins in the spermatic cord due to incompetent valves within the vein, which permit reflux of blood. Most often on left side, perhaps because left spermatic vein is longer and inserts at a right angle into left renal vein. Common in young males. Screen at early adolescence; early treatment important to prevent potential infertility when an adult. Treatment is relatively easy; surgical ligation of spermatic vein.

TABLE 17–1	Abnormalities in the Scrotum—(cont'd)	
Disorder	Clinical Findings	Discussion
Spermatocele	S: Painless, usually found on examination O: Inspection—does transilluminate higher in the scrotum than a hydrocele, and the sperm may fluoresce Palpation—round, freely movable mass lying above and behind testis. If large, feels like a third testis A: Free cystic mass on epididymis	Retention cyst in epididymis. Cause unclear but may be obstruction of tubules. Filled with thin, milky fluid that contains sperm. Most spermatoceles are small (<1 cm); occasionally, they may be larger and then mistaken for hydrocele.
Early Testicular Tumor	S: Painless, found on examination O: Palpation—firm nodule or harder than normal section of testicle A: Solitary nodule	Most testicular tumors occur between the ages of 18 and 35. Practically all are malignant. Occur in whites; relatively rare in blacks, Mexican-Americans, and Asians. Must biopsy to confirm. Most important risk factor is undescended testis, even those surgically corrected. Early detection important in prognosis, but practice of testicular self-examination is currently low.
Diffuse Tumor	S: Enlarging testis (most common symptom). When enlarges, has feel of increased weight O: Inspection—enlarged, does not transilluminate Palpation—enlarged, smooth, ovoid, firm. Important—firm palpation does not cause usual sickening discomfort as with normal testis A: Nontender swelling of testis	Diffuse tumor maintains shape of testis.

Illustrations © Pat Thomas, 2006.

TABLE 17–1	Abnormalities in the Scrotum—(cont'd)	
Disorder	Clinical Findings	Discussion
Hydrocele	S: Painless swelling, although person may complain of weight and bulk in scrotum O: Inspection—enlarged, mass does transilluminate with a pink or red glow (in contrast to a hernia) Palpation—nontender mass, able to get fingers above mass (in contrast to scrotal hernia) A: Nontender swelling of testis	Cystic. Circumscribed collection of serous fluid in tunica vaginalis, surrounding testis. May occur following epididymitis, trauma, hernia, tumor of testis, or spontaneously in the newborn.
Scrotal Hernia	S: Swelling, may have pain with straining O: Inspection—enlarged, may reduce when supine, does not transilluminate Palpation—soft mushy mass, palpating fingers cannot get above mass. Mass is distinct from testicle that is normal A: Nontender swelling of scrotum	Scrotal hernia usually due to indirect inguinal hernia.
Orchitis	S: Acute or moderate pain of sudden onset, swollen testis, feeling of weight, fever O: Inspection—enlarged, edematous, reddened; does not transilluminate Palpation—swollen, congested, tense, and tender; hard to distinguish testis from epididymis A: Tender swelling of testis	Acute inflammation of testis. Most common cause is mumps; can occur with any infectious disease. May have associated hydrocele that does transilluminate.

Illustrations © Pat Thomas, 2006.

TABLE 17–1	Abnormalities in the Scrotum—(cont'd)	
Disorder	Clinical Findings	Discussion
Sctoral Edema	S: Tenderness O: Inspection—enlarged, may be reddened (with local irritation) Palpation—taut with pitting Probably unable to feel scrotal contents A: Scrotal edema	Accompanies marked edema in lower half of body, e.g., congestive heart failure, renal failure, and portal vein obstruction. Occurs with local inflammation: epididymitis, torsion of spermatic cord. Also obstruction of inguinal lymphatics produces lymphedema of scrotum.

Illustrations © Pat Thomas, 2006.

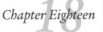

Chapter Eighteen

Female Genitourinary System

ANATOMY

EXTERNAL GENITALIA

The external genitalia are called the **vulva** or pudendum (Fig. 18–1). The **mons pubis** is a round, firm pad of adipose tissue covering the symphysis pubis. The labia majora and labia minora encircle a space termed the **vestibule.** Within this space, the urethral meatus appears as a dimple 2.5 cm posterior to the clitoris. The **clitoris** is a small, pea-shaped erectile body that is highly sensitive to tactile stimulation.

The vaginal orifice is posterior to the urethral meatus. On either side and posterior to the vaginal orifice are the two **Bartholin's glands,** which secrete a clear lubricating mucus during intercourse.

INTERNAL GENITALIA

The **vagina** is a flattened tubular canal extending from the orifice up and backward into the pelvis (Fig. 18–2). At the end of the canal, the uterine **cervix** projects into the vagina.

The **uterus** is a pear-shaped, thick-walled, muscular organ. It is

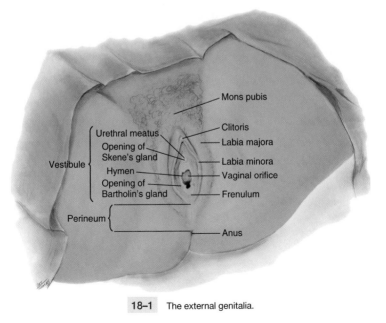

18–1   The external genitalia.

ANTERIOR VIEW OF ADNEXA

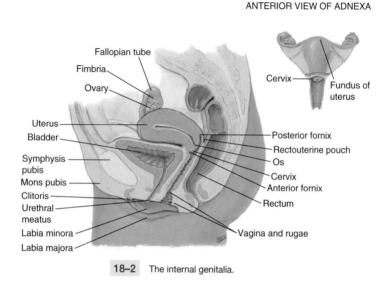

18–2   The internal genitalia.

flattened anteroposteriorly, measuring 5.5 to 8 cm long by 3.5 to 4 cm wide and 2 to 2.5 cm thick, and is movable.

The **fallopian tubes** are two trumpet-shaped, pliable tubes, 10 cm in length, extending from the uterine fundus laterally to the brim of the pelvis, with their ends near the ovaries. Each **ovary** is oval, 3 cm long by 2 cm wide by 1 cm thick, and serves to develop ova (eggs) as well as the female hormones.

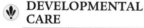 **DEVELOPMENTAL CARE**

The first signs of puberty are breast and pubic hair development, beginning between the ages of $8\frac{1}{2}$ and 13 years. These signs are usually concurrent, but it is not abnormal if they do not develop together. They take about 3 years to complete.

Menarche occurs during the latter half of this sequence, just after the peak of growth velocity.

Tanner's table on the five stages of pubic hair development is helpful in teaching girls the expected sequence of sexual development.

TABLE 18–1	Sex Maturity Rating (SMR) in Girls	
Stage	**Description**	
1	Preadolescent. No pubic hair. Mons and labia covered with fine vellus hair as on abdomen.	
2	Growth sparse and mostly on labia. Long, downy hair, slightly pigmented, straight or only slightly curly.	
3	Growth sparse and spreading over mons pubis. Hair is darker, coarser, curlier.	
4	Hair is adult in type but over smaller area: none on medial thigh.	
5	Adult in type and pattern; inverse triangle. Also on medial thigh surface.	

Adapted from Tanner JM: *Growth at adolescence,* Oxford, England, 1962, Blackwell Scientific.

SUBJECTIVE DATA

1. Menstrual history
   Last menstrual period (LMP)
   Age at menarche
   Cycle
   Duration
2. Obstetric history
   Gravida—number of pregnancies
   Para—number of births
   Abortions—interrupted pregnancies, including elective abortions and spontaneous miscarriages
3. Self-care behaviors
   Gynecologic checkup, Pap smear
4. Urinary symptoms
   Frequency, urgency, dysuria
5. Vaginal discharge—color, characteristics
6. Sexual activity
7. Contraceptive use, condom use
8. Sexually transmitted disease (STD) contact
9. STD risk reduction taught

OBJECTIVE DATA

PREPARATION

Initially, for the health history, the woman should be sitting up.

For the examination, the woman should be placed in the lithotomy position, with the examiner sitting on a stool. Help her into the lithotomy position, with the body supine, feet in stirrups and knees apart, and buttocks at edge of examining table. The arms should be at the woman's sides or across the chest, not over the head, because this position only tightens the abdominal muscles.

Drape the woman fully, covering the stomach, knees, and legs, exposing only the vulva to your view. Be sure to push down the drape between the woman's legs so that you can see her face.

You can help the woman relax, decrease her anxiety, and retain a sense of control by employing these measures.

- Have her empty the bladder before the examination.
- Elevate her head and shoulders to maintain eye contact.
- Place the stirrups so the legs are not abducted too far.
- Explain each step in the examination before you do it.
- Assure the woman she can stop the examination at any point should she feel any discomfort.
- Use a gentle, firm touch with gradual movements.
- Communicate throughout the examination. Maintain a dialog to share information.

EQUIPMENT NEEDED

Assemble these items before helping the woman into position. Arrange within easy reach.

Gloves—wear gloves during every female genitalia examination

Goose-necked lamp with a strong light

Vaginal speculum of appropriate size
   Graves' speculum—useful for adult women, available in varying lengths and widths
   Pedersen speculum—narrow blades useful for young or post-menopausal women with a narrowed introitus

Large cotton-tipped applicators (rectal swabs)

Materials for cytologic study:
   Glass slide with frosted end
   Endocervical brush (cytobrush) or sterile cotton-tipped applicator
   Ayre spatula
   Spray fixative
   Specimen container for gonococcus/chlamydia

Lubricant

Normal Range of Findings	Abnormal Findings

Inspect the External Genitalia

Note:
- Skin color
- Hair distribution is in the usual female pattern of inverted triangle, although it may normally trail up the abdomen toward the umbilicus.
- Labia majora are normally symmetric, plump, and well formed. In the nulliparous woman, labia meet in the midline; following a vaginal delivery, the labia are gaping and slightly shriveled.
- There should be no lesions, except for occasional sebaceous cysts. These are yellowish, 1-cm nodules that are firm, nontender, and often multiple.

With your gloved hand, separate the labia majora to inspect:
- Clitoris
- Labia minora are dark pink and moist, usually symmetric.
- Urethral opening appears stellate or slitlike and is midline.
- Vaginal opening, or introitus, may appear as a narrow vertical slit or as a larger opening.
- Perineum is smooth. A well-healed episiotomy scar, midline or mediolateral, may be present after a vaginal birth.
- Anus has coarse skin of increased pigmentation (see Chapter 19 for assessment).

Palpate Glands

Assess urethra and Skene's glands. Insert your index finger into the vagina, and gently milk the urethra by applying pressure up and out. This procedure should produce no pain. If any discharge appears, culture it.

Assess Bartholin's glands. Palpate the posterior parts of the labia majora

Abnormal Findings (right column)

Consider delayed puberty if no pubic hair or breast development has occurred by age 13.
Nits or lice at the base of pubic hair.
Swelling.

Excoriation. Nodules. Rash/lesions. Refer suspicious red, white, or pigmented lesion for evaluation and biopsy (see Table 26–2, p. 784, in Jarvis: *Physical Examination and Health Assessment,* 5th ed.).

Enlarged clitoris.
Inflammation.

Polyp.

Rash or lesions.
Foul-smelling; irritating; or yellow, white, or gray discharge.

Tenderness.

Induration along urethra.

Urethral discharge.

Swelling.

Normal Range of Findings	Abnormal Findings
with your index finger in the vagina and your thumb outside (Fig. 18–3). The labia normally feel soft and homogeneous.	Pain on palpation. Discharge from duct opening.

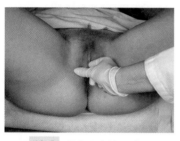

18–3   Palpate labia majora.

Assess the Support of Pelvic Musculature

• Palpate the perineum. It normally feels thick, smooth, and muscular in nulliparous women and thin and rigid in multiparous women.	Tenderness. Paper-thin perineum.
• Using your index and middle fingers, separate the vaginal orifice and ask the woman to strain down. There normally is no bulging of vaginal walls or urinary incontinence.	Bulging of the vaginal wall indicates cystocele, rectocele, or uterine prolapse (see Table 26–3, p. 786, in Jarvis: *Physical Examination and Health Assessment,* 5th ed.). Urinary incontinence.

Internal Genitalia

Speculum Examination

Select the proper-sized speculum. Warm and lubricate the speculum under warm, running water. Avoid gel lubricant at this point because it is bacteriostatic and would distort cells in the cytology specimen you will collect.

Hold the speculum in your left hand with the index and the middle fingers surrounding the blades and your thumb under the thumbscrew. This prevents the blades from opening painfully during insertion. With

Normal Range of Findings	Abnormal Findings

your right index and middle fingers, push the introitus down and open to relax the pubococcygeal muscle (Fig. 18–4).

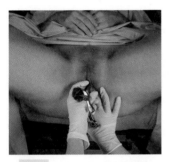

18–4   Invert vaginal speculum.

Tilt the width of the blades obliquely, and insert the speculum past your right fingers, applying any pressure downward. This avoids pressure on the anterior vaginal wall and on the sensitive urethra above it.

Ease insertion by asking the woman to bear down. This method relaxes the perineal muscles and opens the introitus.

As the blades pass your right fingers, withdraw your fingers. Now change the hand holding the speculum to your right hand, and turn the width of the blades horizontally. Continue to insert in a 45-degree angle downward toward the small of the woman's back. This matches the natural slope of the vagina.

After the blades are fully inserted, open them by squeezing the handles together (Fig. 18–5). The cervix should be in full view. Lock the blades open by tightening the thumbscrew.

Abnormal Findings

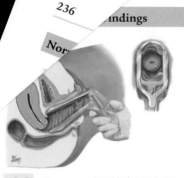

18–5 Open speculum blades and view cervix.

Inspect the Cervix and Its Os

Note:
- Color—Normally, the cervical mucosa is pink and even. During the second month of pregnancy it looks blue (Chadwick's sign), and after menopause it is pale.

- Position—Midline, either anterior or posterior. It projects 1 to 3 cm into the vagina.

- Size—Diameter is 2.5 cm (1 inch).

- Os—Small and round in nulliparous women. In parous women, it is a horizontal irregular slit and may show healed lacerations on the sides.

- Surface—Normally smooth.

- Cervical secretions—Depending on the day of the menstrual cycle, secretions may be clear and thin or thick, opaque, and stringy. They are always odorless and nonirritating.

If secretions are copious, swab the area with a thick-tipped rectal swab. This method sponges away secretions, giving you a better view of the structures.

Redness, inflammation.
Pallor with anemia.
Cyanosis other than with pregnancy.
(See Table 26–4, p. 787, in Jarvis: *Physical Examination and Health Assessment,* 5th ed.)

Surface reddened, granular and any lesion (see erosion, polyp, carcinoma, Table 26–4, p. 787, in Jarvis: *Physical Examination and Health Assessment,* 5th ed.).

Foul-smelling; irritating; or yellow, green, white, or gray discharge (see Table 26–5, p. 789, in Jarvis: *Physical Examination and Health Assessment,* 5th ed.).

Normal Range of Findings	Abnormal Findings

Obtain Cervical Smears and Cultures

The Papanicolaou (Pap) smear screens for cervical cancer. Instruct the woman not to douche or have intercourse within 24 hours before collecting the specimens. The test requires three specimens:

Vaginal Pool. Gently rub the blunt end of an Ayre spatula over the vaginal wall under and lateral to the cervix (Fig. 18-6). Wipe the specimen on a slide and spray with fixative immediately. If the mucosa is very dry (as in a postmenopausal woman), moisten a sterile swab with normal saline to collect this specimen.

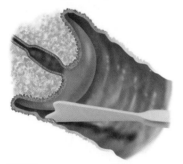

18–6 Pap smear specimens: vaginal pool.

Cervical Scrape. Insert the notched end of an Ayre spatula into the cervical os (Fig. 18-7). Rotate it 360 to 720 degrees, using firm pressure. The spatula scrapes the surface of the cervix as you turn the instrument. Spread the specimen from both sides of the spatula onto a glass slide. Use a single stroke to thin out the specimen, not a back-and-forth motion.

Endocervical Smear. Insert a cytobrush into the os, and rotate it 720 degrees in ONE direction (Fig. 18-8). Then rotate the brush gently on a glass slide to deposit all the cells.

ndings	**Abnormal Findings**

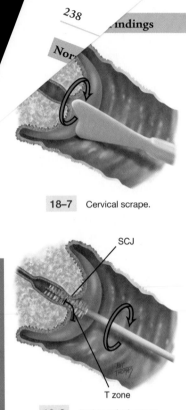

18–7 Cervical scrape.

SCJ

T zone

18–8 Endocervical smear.

Rotate in the opposite direction from the one in which you obtained the specimen. Avoid leaving a thick specimen that would be hard to read under the microscope. Immediately (within 2 seconds) spray all slides with fixative to avoid drying.

Inspect the Vaginal Wall

Loosen the thumbscrew but continue to hold the speculum blades open. Slowly withdraw the speculum, rotating it as you go, to fully inspect the vaginal wall. Normally, the wall looks pink, deeply rugated, moist, and smooth, and it is free of inflammation or lesions. Normal discharge is thin and clear or opaque and stringy, but always is odorless.

Reddened.

Pallor prior to menopause.

Lesions; refer any suspicious red, white, or pigmented lesion for biopsy.

Vaginal discharge—thick, any gray, green-yellow, white, or foul-smelling discharge.

(See Table 26–5, p. 789, in Jarvis: *Physical Examination and Health Assessment,* 5th ed.)

Normal Range of Findings	Abnormal Findings
When the blade ends near the vaginal opening, let them close, but be careful not to pinch the mucosa or catch any hairs. Turn the blades obliquely to avoid stretching the opening. Clean the metal speculum, and place it in a sterilizing and disinfecting solution; discard the plastic variety. Discard your gloves and wash hands.	

Bimanual Examination

Rise to a stand, and have the woman remain in the lithotomy position. Glove and lubricate the first two fingers of your intravaginal hand. Insert your fingers into the vagina, with any pressure directed posteriorly.

Use both hands to palpate the internal genitalia to assess their location, size, and mobility and to screen for any tenderness or mass. One hand is on the abdomen while the other (often the dominant, more sensitive hand) inserts two fingers into the vagina.

Palpate the Internal Genitalia

Normal Range of Findings	Abnormal Findings
Palpate the vaginal wall. It normally feels smooth and has no area of induration or tenderness.	Nodule. Tenderness.
Locate the cervix in the midline, often near the anterior vaginal wall. Note these characteristics of a normal cervix:	
• Consistency—Feels smooth and firm, as the consistency of the tip of the nose. It softens and feels velvety at 5 to 6 weeks of pregnancy (Goodell's sign).	Hard with malignancy. Nodular.
• Contour—Evenly rounded.	Irregular.
• Mobility—With a finger on either side, move the cervix gently from side to side. Normally, this produces no pain (Fig. 18–9).	Immobile with malignancy. Painful with inflammation or ectopic pregnancy.
Palpate all around the fornices; the wall should feel smooth.	Nodular. Irregular.

Normal Range of Findings	**Abnormal Findings**

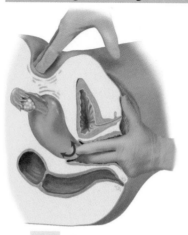

18–9   Palpate the cervix.

Next, use your abdominal hand to push the pelvic organs closer for your intravaginal fingers to palpate. Place your hand midway between the umbilicus and the symphysis; push down in a slow, firm manner, with the fingers together and slightly flexed.

With your intravaginal fingers in the anterior fornix, assess the uterus. Determine the position, or *version,* of the uterus. In many women, the uterus is anteverted; you palpate it at the level of the pubis with the cervix pointing posteriorly. Two other positions normally occur (midposition and retroverted), as well as two aspects of flexion, where the long axis of the uterus is not straight but flexed (for illustration, see Fig. 26–20, p. XXX, in Jarvis: *Physical Examination and Health Assessment,* 5th ed.).

Palpate the uterine wall with your fingers in the fornices. It normally feels firm and smooth, with the contour of the fundus rounded. It softens during pregnancy. Bounce the uterus gently between your abdominal and intravaginal hand. It should be freely movable and nontender.

Enlarged uterus (see Table 26–6, p. 790, in Jarvis: *Physical Examination and Health Assessment,* 5th ed.).

Lateral displacement.

Nodular mass. Irregular, asymmetric. Fixed.

Tenderness.

Normal Range of Findings	Abnormal Findings

Move both hands to the right to explore the adnexa. Place your abdominal hand on the lower quadrant just inside the anterior iliac spine with your intravaginal fingers in the lateral fornix (Fig. 18–10). Push the abdominal hand in and try to capture the ovary. You often cannot feel the ovary. When you can, it normally feels smooth, firm, and almond-shaped; it is highly movable, sliding through the fingers. It is slightly sensitive but not painful. The fallopian tube is not normally palpable. There should be no other mass or pulsation.

Enlarged adnexa.
Nodular.
Immobile.
Markedly tender.
Mass.

Pulsation or a palpable fallopian tube suggests ectopic pregnancy and warrants immediate referral (see Table 26–7, p. 791, in Jarvis: *Physical Examination and Health Assessment*, 5th ed.).

A note of caution: Normal adnexal structures are often not palpable. To be safe, any mass that you cannot *positively* identify as a normal structure should be considered abnormal, and the woman should be referred for further study.

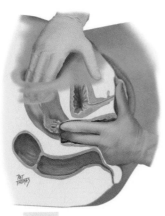

18–10   Palpate the adnexa.

Move to the left to palpate the other side. Then withdraw your hand and check secretions on the fingers before discarding the glove. Normal secretions are clear or cloudy and odorless.

Rectovaginal Examination

Use this technique to assess the rectovaginal septum, posterior uterine wall, cul-de-sac, and rectum. Lubricate your first two fingers. Tell the woman this may feel uncomfortable

Normal Range of Findings	Abnormal Findings

and will mimic the feeling of moving her bowels. Ask her to bear down as you inser your index finger into the vagina and your middle finger gently into the rectum (Fig. 18–11).

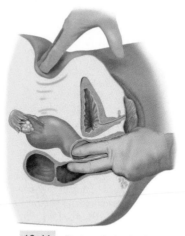

18–11   Rectovaginal palpation.

While pushing with the abdominal hand, repeat the steps of the bimanual examination. Try to keep the intravaginal finger on the cervix so the intrarectal finger does not mistake the cervix for a mass. Note:

- Rectovaginal septum should feel smooth, thin, firm, and pliable.
- Rectovaginal pouch, or cul-de-sac, is a potential space and usually not palpated.
- Uterine wall and fundus feel firm and smooth.

Rotate the intrarectal finger to check the rectal wall and anal sphincter tone. (See Chapter 19 for assessment of the anus and rectum.) Check your gloved finger as you withdraw; test any adherent stool for occult blood.

Give the woman tissues to wipe the area and help her up. Remind her to slide her hips back from the table

Nodular.
Thickened.

Normal Range of Findings	Abnormal Findings
edge before sitting up so she does not fall.	

☙ DEVELOPMENTAL CARE

The Pregnant Female

The external genitalia show hyperemia of the perineum and vulva because of increased vascularity. Varicose veins may be visible in the labia or legs. Hemorrhoids may show around the anus. Both are caused by interruption in venous return from the pressure of the fetus.

Internally, the walls of the vagina appear violet or blue because of hyperemia. The vaginal walls are deeply rugated, and the vaginal mucosa is thickened. The cervix looks blue and feels velvety and softer than in the nonpregnant state, making it a bit more difficult to differentiate from the vaginal walls.

During bimanual examination, the isthmus of the uterus feels softer and is more easily compressed between your two hands (Hegar's sign). The fundus balloons between your two hands: it feels connected to, but distinct from, the cervix because the isthmus is so soft.

Search the adnexal area carefully during early pregnancy. Normally, the adnexal structures are not palpable.

An ectopic pregnancy has serious consequences (see Table 26–7, p. 791, in Jarvis: *Physical Examination and Health Assessment,* 5th ed.).

The Aging Adult

Natural lubrication is decreased; to avoid a painful examination, take care to lubricate instruments and the examining hand adequately. Use the Pedersen speculum with its narrower, flatter blades.

Menopause and the resulting decrease in estrogen production cause numerous physical changes. Pubic

Normal Range of Findings	Abnormal Findings
hair gradually decreases, becoming thin and sparse in later years. Fat deposits decrease, leaving the mons pubis smaller and the labia flatter. Clitoris size also decreases after age 60. Internally, the rugae of the vaginal walls decrease, and the walls look pale pink because of the thinned epithelium. The cervix shrinks and looks pale and glistening. It may retract, appearing to be flush with the vaginal wall. In some older women, it is hard to distinguish the cervix from the surrounding vaginal mucosa. Alternately, the cervix may protrude into the vagina if the uterus has prolapsed. With the bimanual examination, the uterus feels smaller and firmer, and the ovaries are not normally palpable.	

Summary Checklist

For a PDA-downloadable version go to http://evolve.elsevier.com/Jarvis.

1. Inspect external genitalia
2. Palpate labia and Skene's and Bartholin's glands
3. Using vaginal speculum, inspect cervix and vagina
4. Obtain specimens for cytologic study
5. Perform bimanual examination: cervix, uterus, adnexa
6. Perform rectovaginal examination
7. Test stool for occult blood

Nursing Diagnoses Commonly Associated with the Eyes and Visual Disorders

Delayed **Growth** and development
Functional **Incontinence**
Reflex **Incontinence**
Stress **Incontinence**
Total **Incontinence**
Urge **Incontinence**

Pain
Rape trauma syndrome
Sexual dysfunction
Ineffective **Sexuality** patterns
Impaired **Skin** integrity

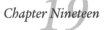

Chapter Nineteen

Anus, Rectum, and Prostate

ANATOMY

The **anal canal** is the outlet of the gastrointestinal tract and is about 3.8 cm long in adults (Fig. 19–1). It slants forward toward the umbilicus, forming a distinct right angle with the rectum, which rests back in the hollow of the sacrum.

The anal canal is surrounded by two concentric layers of muscle: the *internal* and *external sphincters.*

The **rectum,** which is 12 cm long, is the distal portion of the large intestine. Just above the anal canal, the rectum dilates and turns posteriorly, forming the rectal ampulla.

In males, the **prostate gland** lies in front of the anterior wall of the rectum. It surrounds the bladder neck and the urethra, and it secretes a thin, milky alkaline fluid that helps sperm viability. It has two lobes that are separated by a shallow groove called the **median sulcus.** The two **seminal vesicles** project like rabbit ears above the prostate. They secrete a fluid containing fructose, which nourishes the sperm.

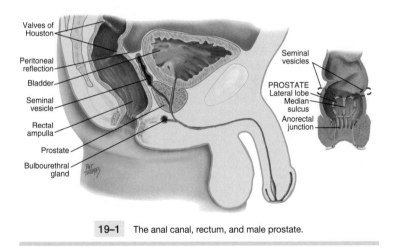

19–1 The anal canal, rectum, and male prostate.

SUBJECTIVE DATA

1. Usual bowel routine: frequency, stool color
2. Change in bowel habits: diarrhea, constipation, use of enemas
3. Rectal bleeding, blood in the stool
4. Medications: laxatives, stool softeners, iron
5. Rectal conditions (pruritus, hemorrhoids, fissure, fistula)
6. Family history: colon, rectal, prostate cancer; polyps; inflammatory bowel disease
7. Diet of high-fiber foods
8. Most recent examinations: digital rectal examination, stool blood test, colonoscopy, prostate-specific antigen blood test (for men)

OBJECTIVE DATA

PREPARATION

Examine the male in the left lateral decutibus position or standing and leaning over an examination table. Place the female in the lithotomy position if examining the genital as well; use the left lateral decubitus position for the rectal area alone.

EQUIPMENT NEEDED

Penlight
Lubricating jelly
Glove
Fecal occult blood test materials

Normal Range of Findings	Abnormal Findings
Inspect the Perianal Area	
The anus normally appears moist and hairless, with coarse, folded, pigmented skin. The anal opening is tightly closed. There are no lesions.	Inflammation. Lesions or scars. Linear split—tissue. Flabby skin sac—hemorrhoid. Shiny blue skin sac—thrombosed hemorrhoid. Small round opening in anal area—fistula.
The sacrococcygeal area appears smooth and even.	Inflammation or tenderness, swelling, a tuft of hair, or a dimple at the tip of the coccyx may indicate pilonidal cyst (see Table 25–1, p. 752, in Jarvis: *Physical Examination and Health Assessment,* 5th ed.).
Instruct the person to hold his or her breath and bear down by performing a Valsalva maneuver. There should be no break in skin integrity or protrusion through the anal opening.	Appearance of fissure or hemorrhoids. Circular red doughnut of tissue—rectal prolapse.

Normal Range of Findings	Abnormal Findings

Palpate the Anus and Rectum

Drop lubricating jelly onto your gloved index finger. Inform the person that palpation is not painful but may feel as if he or she needs to move the bowels.

Place the pad of your index finger gently against the anal verge. You will feel the sphincter tighten, then relax. As it relaxes, flex the tip of your finger and slowly insert it into the anal canal in a direction toward the umbilicus.

Rotate your examining finger to palpate the entire muscular ring. The canal should feel smooth and even. To assess tone, ask the person to tighten the muscle. The sphincter should tighten evenly around your finger with no pain to the person.

Decreased tone.

Increased tone occurs with inflammation and anxiety.

Above the anal canal, the rectum turns posteriorly, following the curve of the coccyx and sacrum. Insert your finger farther and explore all around the rectal wall. It normally feels smooth with no nodularity. Promptly report any mass you discover for further examination.

Thrombosed internal hemorrhoid.

A soft, slightly movable mass may be a polyp.

A firm or hard mass with irregular shape or rolled edges may signify carcinoma (see Table 25–2, p. 754, in Jarvis: *Physical Examination and Health Assessment,* 5th ed.).

Palpate the Prostate Gland

In males, palpate the prostate gland on the anterior wall (Fig. 19–2). Carefully press *into* the gland at each location. Note:
- Size—2.5 cm long by 4 cm wide; should not protrude more than 1 cm into the rectum
- Shape—heart shaped, with palpable central groove
- Surface—smooth
- Consistency—elastic, rubbery
- Mobility—slightly movable
- Sensitivity—nontender to palpation.

Enlarged, or atrophied, gland.

Flat with no groove.

Nodular.

Hard; or boggy, soft, flactuant.

Fixed.

Tender.

Normal Range of Findings	Abnormal Findings

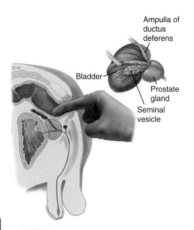

Ampulla of ductus deferens

Bladder

Prostate gland

Seminal vesicle

19–2   Palpate the prostate gland.

Withdraw your examining finger; normally, there is no bright red blood or mucus on the glove. Offer the person tissues to remove the lubricant, and help him or her to a more comfortable position.

Examination of Stool. Inspect any feces remaining on the glove. Normally, the color is brown and the consistency is soft.

Enlarged, firm, smooth gland with obliterated central groove suggests benign prostatic hypertrophy (BPH).

Swollen, exquisitely tender gland accompanied prostatitis.

Any stone-hard, irregular, fixed nodule indicates carcinoma (see Table 25–3, p. 755, in Jarvis: *Physical Examination and Health Assessment,* 5th ed.).

Jelly-like mucus shreds mixed in stool indicate inflammation.

Bright red blood on stool surface indicates rectal bleeding. Bright red blood mixed with feces indicates possible colonic bleeding.

Normal Range of Findings	Abnormal Findings
Test any stool on the glove for *occult* (or hidden) *blood.* Use the *guaiac-impregnated cards* to detect small quantities of blood. A negative response is normal. If the stool is *guaiac positive,* it indicates occult blood. Note that a false-positive finding may occur if the person has ingested significant amounts of red meat within 3 days of the test.	Black, tarry stool with distinct malodor indicates uppr gastrointestinal bleeding, with blood partially digested.

Black stool also occurs with ingesting iron medications or bismuth preparations.

Gray, tan stool occurs with absent bile pigment, e.g., obstructive jaundice.

Pale yellow, greasy stool occurs with increased fat contant (steatorrhea), as occurs with malabsorption syndrome.

Occult bleeding usually indicates cancer of colon. |

Summary Checklist

For a PDA-downloadable version go to http://evolve.elsevier.com/Jarvis.

1. Inspect anus and perianal area
2. Inspect during Valsalva maneuver
3. Palpate anal canal and rectum on all adults
4. Test stool for occult blood

Chapter Twenty

Integration of the Complete Physical Examination

◆——— ANATOMY ———◆

The following examination sequence combines all the separate steps into a complete and smoothly flowing assessment. The sequence clusters steps by body region and proceeds systematically head to toe, concluding with examination of the genitalia. This is the most efficient way of conducting the examination, and it minimizes the number of position changes for you and the patient, thus avoiding tiring the patient. The running second column presents a sample recording when findings are within the normal range.

◆——— OBJECTIVE DATA ———◆

Sequence	Sample Recording
The patient walks into the room and sits; the examiner sits facing the patient; the patient is in street clothes.	

The Health History

1. Collect the history, complete or limited as visit warrants. While obtaining the history and throughout the examination, note data on the person's general appearance.

General Appearance

1. Appears stated age
2. Level of consciousness
3. Skin color
4. Nutritional status
5. Posture and position comfortably erect
6. Obvious physical deformities

(Patient's name) is a (age)-year-old (male/female), well nourished, well developed, who appears stated age. (S)he is alert, oriented, cooperative, with no signs of acute distress. Appearance, behavior, and speech are appropriate; recent and remote memory intact.

The following lined rules indicate position change for examiner or patient.

Sequence	Sample Recording

7. Mobility:
   Gait
   Use of assistive devices
   Range of motion of joints
   No involuntary movement
8. Facial expression
9. Mood and affect
10. Speech:
    Articulation
    Pattern
    Content appropriate
    Native language
11. Hearing
12. Personal hygiene

Measurement

1. Weight
2. Height
3. Compute Body Mass Index
4. Vision using Snellen eye chart

Weight 57 kg (126 lb), height 163 cm (5'4"), skinfold thickness 20 mm, vision OD 20/20, OS 20/30 − 1.

Ask the patient to empty the bladder (save specimen, if needed), to disrobe except for underpants, and to put on a gown. The patient sits with the legs dangling off the side of the bed or table; examiner stands in front of the person.

Skin

1. Examine both hands and inspect the nails.

Skin: Color tan-pink (light brown, brown, brown-black), warm to touch; turgor good, no lesions.

2. For the rest of the examination, examine skin with corresponding regional examination.

Nails: No clubbing or deformities, nail beds pink with prompt capillary refill.

Vital Signs

1. Radial pulse
2. Respirations
3. Blood pressure
4. Temperature
5. Pain assessment

TPR: 37° C–76–14, BP 128/84 right arm, sitting.
Reports no areas of pain.

Head and Face

1. Inspect and palpate scalp, hair, and cranium.

Hair: Texture fine, distribution appropriate for age.

Sequence	Sample Recording

2. Inspect face: expression, symmetry (cranial nerve VII).
3. Palpate the temporal artery, then the temporomandibular joint as the person opens and closes the mouth.
4. Palpate the maxillary sinuses and the frontal sinuses; if tender, transilluminate the sinuses.

Head: Normocephalic, no lumps, no lesions, no tenderness.
Face: Symmetric, no weakness, no involuntary movements.

Eyes

1. Test visual fields by confrontation (cranial nerve II).
2. Test extraocular muscles: corneal light reflex, six cardinal positions of gaze (cranial nerves III, IV, VI).
3. Inspect external eye structures.
4. Inspect conjunctivae, sclerae, corneae, irides.
5. Test pupils: size, response to light and accommodation.

Darken room.

6. Using an ophthalmoscope, inspect ocular fundus: red reflex, disc, vessels, and retinal background.

Eyes: Visual fields intact by confrontation. EOMs intact. Brows and lashes present. No ptosis. Conjunctivae clear. Sclerae white, no lesions. PERRLA.
Fundi: Red reflex present bilaterally. Discs flat with sharp margins. Vessels present in all quadrants without crossing defects. Retinal background has even color with no hemorrhages or exudates. Macula has even color.

Ears

1. Inspect the external ear: position and alignment, skin condition, and auditory meatus.
2. Move auricle and push tragus for tenderness.
3. Using an otoscope, inspect the canal and then the tympanic membrane for color, position, landmarks, and integrity.
4. Test hearing: voice test, tuning fork tests (Weber and Rinne).

Ears: No masses, lesions, tenderness, or discharge. Both TMs pearly gray with light reflex and landmarks intact, no perforations. Whispered words heard bilaterally. Weber test is midline without lateralization. Rinne AC > BC and = bilaterally.

Nose

1. Inspect the external nose: symmetry, lesions.
2. Test the patency of each nostril.

Nose: No deformity. Nares patent. Mucosa pink; no septal deviation or perforation.

Sequence	Sample Recording
3. Using a nasal speculum, inspect the nares: nasal mucosa, septum, and turbinates.	

Mouth and Throat

1. Using a penlight, inspect the mouth: buccal mucosa, teeth and gums, tongue, floor of mouth, palate, and uvula.
2. Grade tonsils, if present.
3. Note mobility of uvula as the person phonates "ahh," and test gag reflex (cranial nerves IX, X).
4. Ask the person to stick out the tongue (cranial nerve XII).
5. Palpate the mouth bimanually if indicated.

Mouth: Can clench teeth. Mucosa and gingivae pink, no masses or lesions. Teeth in good repair. Tongue protrudes in midline; no tremor.

Throat: Mucosa pink, no lesions. Uvula arises in midline on phonation. Tonsils out. Gag reflex present.

Neck

1. Inspect the neck: symmetry, lumps, and pulsations.
2. Palpate the cervical lymph nodes.
3. Inspect and palpate the carotid pulse, one side at a time. If indicated, listen for carotid bruits.
4. Palpate the trachea in midline.
5. Test range of motion and muscle strength against your resistance: head forward and back, head turned to each side, and shoulder shrug (cranial nerve XI).

Step behind the person, taking your stethoscope, ruler, and marking pen with you.

6. Palpate thyroid gland.

Open the person's gown to expose all of the back, but leave gown on shoulders and anterior chest.

Neck: Supple with full ROM, no pain. Symmetric, no lymphadenopathy or masses; trachea midline; thyroid not palpable, no bruits. Carotid pulses 2+ and = bilaterally.

Chest, Posterior and Lateral

1. Inspect the posterior chest: configuration of the thoracic cage, skin characteristics, and symmetry of shoulders and muscles.

Chest: AP < transverse diameter. Respirations 16 per minute, relaxed and even. Chest expansion symmet-

Sequence	Sample Recording
2. Palpate: symmetric expansion, tactile fremitus, lumps, or tenderness.	*ric. Tactile fremitus equal bilaterally. Resonant to percussion over lung fields. Diaphragmatic excursion 5 cm and = bilaterally. Breath sounds clear. No adventitious sounds.*
3. Palpate length of spinous processes.	
4. Percuss over all lung fields, noting diaphragmatic excursion.	
5. Percuss costovertebral angle, noting tenderness.	
6. Auscultate breath sounds, and note adventitious sounds.	

Move around to face the patient; the patient remains sitting. At the time for the female breast examination, ask the woman's permission to lift the gown to drape on the shoulders, exposing the anterior chest; for a male, lower the gown to the lap.

Anterior Chest

1. Inspect: respirations and skin characteristics.
2. Palpate: tactile fremitus, lumps, and tenderness.
3. Percuss lung fields.
4. Auscultate breath sounds.

Heart

1. Ask the person to lean forward slightly and exhale briefly; auscultate base of the heart for any murmurs.

(See Sample Recording in HEART section following.)

Upper Extremities

1. Test range of motion and muscle strength of hands, arms, and shoulders.
2. Palpate the epitrochlear nodes.

(See Sample Recording in LOWER EXTREMITIES section following.)

Female Breasts

1. Inspect for symmetry, mobility, and dimpling as the woman lifts arms over the head, pushes the hands on the hips, and leans forward.

Breasts symmetric. No retraction, no nipple discharge, no lesions. Contour and consistency firm and homogeneous. No masses or tenderness. No lymphadenopathy.

Sequence	Sample Recording
2. Inspect supraclavicular and infra-clavicular areas.	

Help the patient to lie supine with the head at a 30- to 45-degree angle. Stand at the person's *right* side. Drape the gown up across shoulders and place an extra sheet across the lower abdomen.

3. Palpate each breast, lifting the same side arm up over head. Include the tail of Spence and areola.
4. Palpate each nipple for discharge.
5. Support the person's arm and palpate the axilla and regional lymph nodes.
6. Teach breast self-examination.

Male Breasts

1. Inspect and palpate while palpating the anterior chest wall.
2. Supporting each arm, palpate the axilla and regional nodes.

Neck Vessels

1. Inspect each side of neck for a jugular venous pulse, turning the person's head slightly to the other side.
2. Estimate the jugular venous pressure, if indicated.

External jugular veins flat.

Heart

1. Inspect the precordium for pulsations and heave (lift).
2. Palpate the apical impulse, and note the location.
3. Palpate the precordium for thrills.
4. Auscultate the apical rate and rhythm.
5. Auscultate with the diaphragm of the stethoscope to study heart sounds, inching from the apex up to the base, or vice versa.
6. Auscultate the heart sounds with the bell of the stethoscope, again inching through all locations.

Precordium: Apical impulse at 5th intercostal space, left midclavicular line. No heave or thrill, rate 68 per minute and rhythm regular, S_1 and S_2 are normal, not diminished or accentuated, no extra sounds, no murmurs.

Sequence	Sample Recording
7. Turn the person over to the left side while again auscultating the apex with the bell.	

The person should be supine, with the bed or table flat; arrange drapes to expose the abdomen from the chest to the pubis.

Abdomen

1. Inspect: contour, symmetry, skin characteristics, umbilicus, and pulsations.
2. Auscultate bowel sounds.
3. Auscultate for vascular sounds over the aorta and renal arteries.
4. Percuss all quadrants.
5. Percuss height of the liver span in right midclavicular line.
6. Percuss the location of the spleen.
7. Palpate: light palpation in all quadrants, then deep palpation in all quadrants.
8. Palpate for liver, for spleen, for kidneys, and for aorta pulsation.
9. Test the abdominal reflexes, if indicated.

Abdomen: Flat, symmetric with no apparent masses. Skin smooth with no striae, scars, or lesions. Bowel sounds present, no bruits. Tympany to percussion in all 4 quadrants. Liver span 8 cm in right midclavicular line; splenic dullness at 10th intercostal space in left midaxillary line. Abdomen soft to palpation, no organomegaly, no masses, no tenderness.

Inguinal Area

1. Palpate each groin for the femoral pulse and the inguinal nodes.

Lift the drape to expose the legs.

Lower Extremities

1. Inspect: symmetry, skin characteristics, and hair distribution.
2. Palpate pulses: popliteal, posterior tibial, and dorsalis pedis.
3. Palpate for temperature and pretibial edema.
4. Separate toes and inspect.
5. Test range of motion and muscle strength: hips, knees, ankles, and feet.

Extremities have pink-tan (brown, brown-black) color with no redness, cyanosis, or any skin lesions. Extremity size symmetric with no swelling or atrophy. Temperature warm and = bilaterally. All pulses present, 2+ and = bilaterally. No lymphadenopathy.

(See MUSCULOSKELETAL section below for muscle sample recording.)

Ask the patient to sit up and dangle the legs off the bed or table. Keep the gown on, and drape it over the lap.

Sequence	Sample Recording

Musculoskeletal

1. Note muscle strength as person performs the sit-up.

Neurologic

Note: Testing of cranial nerves II to XII was integrated during head and neck regional examinations.

1. Test sensation in selected areas on face, arms, hands, legs, and feet: superficial pain, light touch, and vibration.
2. Test position sense of finger, one hand.
3. Test stereognosis.
4. Test cerebellar function of the upper extremities using finger-to-nose test or rapid alternating movements test.
5. Test the cerebellar function of the lower extremities by asking the person to run each heel down the opposite shin.
6. Elicit deep tendon reflexes: biceps, triceps, brachioradialis, patellar, and Achilles.
7. Test the Babinski reflex.

Neurologic, sensory: Pinprick, light touch, vibration intact. Stereognosis—able to identify key.

Motor: No atrophy, weakness, or tremors. RAM (rapid alternating movements)—finger-to-nose smoothly intact.

Reflexes: Normal abdominal, DTRs all 2+ and equal bilaterally, no Babinski sign.

Ask the patient to stand with the gown on. Stand close to the patient.

Lower Extremities

1. Inspect lower legs for varicose veins.

Musculoskeletal

1. Ask the person to walk across the room, turn, then walk back toward you in heel-to-toe fashion.
2. Ask the person to walk on the toes for a few steps, then to walk on the heels for a few steps.
3. Stand close, and check the Romberg sign.

Musculoskeletal: Gait smooth and fluid, able to tandem walk, no Romberg sign. Joints and muscles symmetric; no swelling, masses, or deformity; normal spinal curvature.

Sequence	Sample Recording
4. Ask the person to hold the edge of the bed and to perform a shallow knee bend, one for each leg. 5. Stand behind and check the spine as the person touches the toes. 6. Stabilize the pelvis and test range of motion of the spine as the person hyperextends, rotates, and laterally bends.	*No tenderness to palpation of joints; no heat, swelling, or masses. Full ROM; movement smooth, no crepitance, no tenderness. Muscle strength—able to maintain flexion against resistance and without tenderness.*

Sit on a stool in front of a male patient. The male stands.

Male Genitalia

1. Inspect the penis and scrotum.
2. Palpate the scrotal contents. If a mass exists, transilluminate.
3. Check for inguinal hernia.
4. Teach testicular self-examination.

Male genitalia: No lesions, no inflammation or discharge from penis. Scrotum—testes descended, symmetric, no masses. No inguinal hernia.

For an adult male, ask him to bend over the examination table, supporting the torso with his forearms on the table, and stand with the feet positioned with the toes turned inward. Assist a bedfast male to a left lateral position with his right leg drawn up. The examiner stands.

Male Rectum

1. Inspect the perianal area.
2. With a gloved, lubricated finger, palpate the rectal walls and prostate gland.
3. Save a stool specimen for guaiac test.

Rectum: No fissures, hemorrhoids, fistulas, or skin lesions in perianal area. Sphincter tone good, no prolapse. Rectal walls smooth, no masses or tenderness. Prostate not enlarged, no masses or tenderness. Stool brown, guaiac negative.

For an adult female, assist her back to the examination table and help her assume the lithotomy position. Drape her appropriately. Examiner sits on a stool at the foot of the table, then stands.

Female Genitalia

1. Inspect the perineal and perianal areas.
2. Using a vaginal speculum, inspect the cervix and vaginal walls.
3. Procure specimens.

External genitalia: No swelling, lesions, or discharge. No urethral swelling or discharge. Internal genitalia: Vaginal walls have no bulging or lesions; cervix pink with no le-

Sequence	Sample Recording
4. Perform a bimanual examination: cervix, uterus, and adnexa.	sions, scant clear mucoid discharge. *Bimanual:* No pain on moving cervix; uterus anteflexed and anteverted. *Adnexa:* Ovaries not enlarged.
5. Continue the bimanual examination, checking the rectum and rectovaginal walls.	
6. Save a stool specimen for guaiac test.	*Rectum:* No hemorrhoids, fissures, or lesions; no masses or tenderness. Stool brown, guaiac negative.
7. Wipe the perineal area with tissues, and help her up to a sitting position.	

Tell the person you are finished with the examination and that you will leave the room as he or she gets dressed. Return to discuss the examination and further plans and answer any questions. Thank the person for his or her time.

For the hospitalized patient, return the bed and any room equipment to the way you found it. Make sure the call light and telephone are within easy reach.

Recording the Data

Record the data from the history and physical examination as soon after the event as possible. Memory fades as your day progresses, especially when you are responsible for the care of more than one person.

It is difficult to strike a balance between recording too few data and recording too much. It is important to remember that, from a legal perspective, if it is not documented, it was not done. Data important for the diagnosis and treatment of the person's health should be recorded as well as data that contribute to your decision-making process. This includes charting relevant normal or negative findings.

On the other hand, a listing of every assessment parameter yields an unwieldy, unworkable record. One way to keep your record complete yet succinct is to study your writing style. Use short, clear phrases. Avoid redundant introductory phrases such as, "The patient states that. . . ." Avoid redundant descriptions such as "no

Sequence	Sample Recording
inguinal, femoral, or umbilical hernias." Just write, "no hernias." Use simple line drawings to describe your findings. You do not need artistic talent; draw a simple sketch of a tympanic membrane, breast, abdomen, or cervix and mark your findings on it. A clear picture is worth many sentences.	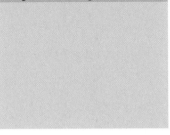

Chapter 4

Figure 4-3: From Brest AM, Moyer JH: *Hypertension: recent advances.* Philadelphia, Lea & Febiger, 1961. Reprinted with permission.

Chapter 7

Figure 7-1: Copyright Pat Thomas, 2006.

Chapter 8

Figure 8-1: Copyright Pat Thomas, 2006.

Chapter 9

Figures 9-1 and 9-2: Copyright Pat Thomas, 2006.

Table 9-1: **Acute Tonsillitis and Pharyngitis:** from Hawke M: *Diagnostic handbook of otorhinolaryngology.* Martin Dunitz, Ltd., 1998; **Cheilitis (Angular Stomatitis, Perleche):** from Callen JP, Greer KE, Hood AF, et al: *Color Atlas of Dermatology,* Philadelphia, W.B. Saunders, 1993, p. 326; **Herpes Simplex I:** from Callen JP, Greer KE, Hood AF, et al: *Color Atlas of Dermatology,* Philadelphia, W.B. Saunders, 1993, p. 168; **Gingivitis:** from Callen JP, Greer KE, Hood AF, et al: *Color Atlas of Dermatology,* W.B. Saunders, 1993, p. 385; **Aphthous Ulcers:** from Sleisinger MH, Fordtran JS: *Gastrointestinal Diseases: Pathophysiology, Diagnosis, and Management,* ed 5, vol 1, Philadelphia, Saunders, 1993, Color plate WVII-B; **Torus Palatinus:** from Ibsen OAC, Phelen JA: *Oral Pathology for the Dental Hygienist,* ed 2, Philadelphia, Saunders, 1996, slide 284.

Chapter 15

Figure 15-9: From Rossman I: *Clinical geriatrics,* 3rd ed. J.B. Lippincott Company, Williams, and Wilkins, 1986, p. 6.

Chapter 16

Figures 16-1, 16-2, and 16-3: Copyright Pat Thomas, 2006.

Figure 16-19: From Hickey JV: *Neurological and neurosurgical nursing,* 2nd ed. Philadelphia, JB Lippincott Company, 1986, p. 121.

Chapter 17

Unnumbered Figures in Table 7-1: Copyright Pat Thomas, 2006.

REFERENCES

American Heart Association: 2007 Heart disease and stroke statistics: www.americanheart.org/downloadable/heart. Accessed February 2007.

American Cancer Society: *What are the risk factors for breast cancer?* Available at http://www.cancer.org/docroot/CRI/content/CRI_2_4_2X_What_are_the_risk_factors_for_breast_cancer_5.asp. Accessed August 2007.

American Pain Society (APS): Principles of analgesic use in the treatment of acute and cancer pain, ed 3, Glenview, IL, 1992.

Beyer JE: *The oucher: A user's manual and technical report.* Evanston, IL, 1983, Judson.

Folstein MF, Folstein SE, McHugh PR: "Mini-Mental State": A practical method for grading the cognitive state of patients for the clinician. J Psychiatr Res 12:189-198, 1975.

Herman-Giddens ME, Slora EJ, Wasserman RC et al: Secondary sexual characteristics and menses in young girls seen in office practice: A study from the pediatric research in office settings network. *Pediatrics* 99(4):505–512, Apr 1997.

Love S, Lindsey K: *Dr. Susan Love's breast book,* 3rd ed, Cambridge, MA, 2000, Perseus Publishing.

McCaffery M: *Nursing practice theories related to cognition, bodily pain, and man-environment interactions,* Los Angeles, 1968, UCLA, Students Store.

Overfield T: *Biologic variation in health and illness: Race, age, and sex differences,* 2nd ed, New York, 1995, CRC Press.

Terris MH, Magit AE, Davidson TE: Otitis media with effusion in infants and children. *Postgrad Med* 97:137-151, 1995.

INDEX